IMAGING IN REHABILITATION

Notice

Medicine is an ever-changing science. As new research and clinical experience broaden our knowledge, changes in treatment and drug therapy are required. The authors and the publisher of this work have checked with sources believed to be reliable in their efforts to provide information that is complete and generally in accord with the standards accepted at the time of publication. However, in view of the possibility of human error or changes in medical sciences, neither the authors nor the publisher nor any other party who has been involved in the preparation or publication of this work warrants that the information contained herein is in every respect accurate or complete, and they disclaim all responsibility for any errors or omissions or for the results obtained from use of the information contained in this work. Readers are encouraged to confirm the information contained herein with other sources. For example and in particular, readers are advised to check the product information sheet included in the package of each drug they plan to administer to be certain that the information contained in this work is accurate and that changes have not been made in the recommended dose or in the contraindications for administration. This recommendation is of particular importance in connection with new or infrequently used drugs.

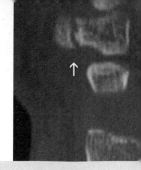

IMAGING IN REHABILITATION

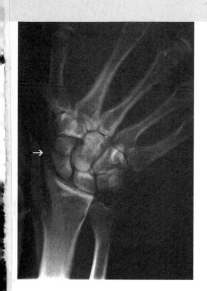

Terry R. Malone, EdD, PT, ATC, FAPTA
Professor, Division of Physical Therapy
College of Health Sciences
Department of Rehabilitation Sciences
University of Kentucky
Lexington, Kentucky

Charles Hazle, PT, MS
Assistant Professor, Division of Physical Therapy
College of Health Sciences
Department of Rehabilitation Sciences
University of Kentucky
Center for Excellence in Rural Health
Hazard, Kentucky

Michael L. Grey, MS, RT(R)(MR)(CT)
Associate Professor
Radiologic Sciences
MRI/CT Specialization
School of Allied Health
College of Applied Sciences and Arts
Southern Illinois University
Carbondale, Illinois

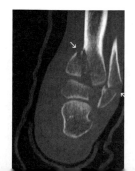

Mc Graw Hill Medical

New York   Chicago   San Francisco   Lisbon   London   Madrid
Mexico City   Milan   New Delhi   San Juan   Seoul
Singapore   Sydney   Toronto

Imaging in Rehabilitation

1 2 3 4 5 6 7 8 9 0   DOC/DOC   0 9 8

Set ISBN 978-0-07-144778-2
Set MHID 0-07-144778-4
Book ISBN 978-0-07-154946-2
Book MHID 0-07-154946-3
CD ISBN 978-0-07-154947-9
CD MHID 0-07-154947-1

This book was set in Frutiger by International Typesetting and Composition.
The editors were Catherine A. Johnson and Christie Naglieri.
The production supervisor was Sherri Souffrance.
Project management was provided by Preeti Longia Sinha, International Typesetting and Composition.
The designer was Cathleen Elliott.
RR Donnelley was printer and binder.

This book is printed on acid-free paper.

INTERNATIONAL EDITION ISBN-13: 978-0-07-128736-4; ISBN-10: 0-07-128736-1

Library of Congress Cataloging-in-Publication Data

Malone, Terry, 1950-
    Imaging in rehabilitation / Terry R. Malone, Charles Hazle, Michael L. Grey.
        p. ; cm.
    Includes index.
    ISBN-13: 978-0-07-144778-2 (pbk. : alk. paper)
    ISBN-10: 0-07-144778-4 (pbk. : alk. paper)
    1. Diagnostic imaging.   2. Musculoskeletal system—Imaging.   3. Physical therapy.
    4. Rehabilitation.   I. Hazle, Charles.   II. Grey, Michael L.   III. Title.
    [DNLM: 1. Diagnostic Imaging.   2. Musculoskeletal Diseases—diagnosis.
    3. Physical Therapy Modalities.   4. Rehabilitation—methods. WN 180 M257i   2008]
    RC78.7.D53M34   2008
    616.07'54—dc22
                                                                        2007036096

DEDICATION

A big thank you to the staff and students of the University of Kentucky—this project would never have been accomplished without your assistance and support—to my wife Becky and sons Matthew and Mark—thanks for your encouragement and love.

TRM

For my parents.

CRH

To my loving wife, Rebecca, and wonderful children, Kayla, Emily and Megan. Thank you for your support and encouragement.

Michael (Dada)

CONTENTS

PREFACE

Imaging has dramatically changed through the recent applications of computer and imaging technologies. Likewise, the last 25 years have seen the physical therapy profession evolve from primarily baccalaureate programs to the present day clinical doctoral degree (Doctor of Physical Therapy). This evolution has included the additional emphasis of physical therapists providing significantly more information to their patients related to the special tests and greatly enhanced imaging study results related to how these results impact the customization of the rehabilitation program. This text was designed to provide the physical therapist and the physical therapy student a user friendly guide to applications of the common imaging modalities and the basic interpretation of these images. Each regional chapter provides the special applications unique to that region and how clinicians can select for optimal clinical decision making. In an attempt to demonstrate this, these chapters have case studies which illustrate concepts in a real world setting. As many users may have a limited previous exposure to imaging, a CD-ROM providing image and contextual information is provided to enhance general appreciation and interpretation. Many readers may use the Asian approach to publication as we have a "Primer of Reading an Image" as the last chapter of the text. Students may begin at the beginning—jump to the end—and then proceed through the regional chapters to best facilitate retention. We hope this text will serve as a useful introduction to the fascinating and exploding world of imaging—serving the student and practicing therapist well.

ACKNOWLEDGMENTS

We wish to offer a special thank you to all the clinicians and their medical staffs for providing us the de-identified imaging studies illustrating the text: University of Kentucky Sports Medicine and Orthopaedics (Drs. Darren Johnson, Scott Mair, Michael Boland, Mauro Giordani, and Robert Hosey): Dr. Juan Yepes (University of Kentucky College of Dentistry): Dr. Sheri Albers (University of Kentucky Department of Radiology), Kentucky Sports Medicine (Dr. Mary Lloyd Ireland), Duke University Sports Medicine (Drs. William Garrett and Claude T. Moorman), Methodist Sports Medicine Center (Drs. John McCarroll, Gary Misamore, and Arthur Rettig), University of Evansville (Dr. Kyle Kiesel), Washington University Medical Center–Mallinckrodt Institute of Radiology (Dr. William D. Middleton), University of Iowa Hospitals and Clinics (Dr. Theodore Donta and Mr. Mark A. Nicklaus, RT (R)(CT), and Dr. Fulk at Cedar Court Imaging, Carbondale, Illinois. We also thank Sheryl Abercrombie and Linda Dalton, University of Kentucky Medical Center Image Management; Dr. Kay-Geert A. Hermann, Department of Radiology, Charité Medical School, Berlin, Germany; and reviewers G. Jeffrey Popham, MD, and Gail Deyle, PT, DSC, DPT.

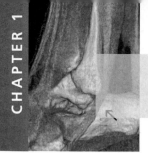
Introduction to Musculoskeletal Imaging

Most musculoskeletal injuries occur as a result of either trauma or overuse. Following a thorough evaluation by a qualified health-care professional, most patients are usually required to have a basic radiographic (x-ray) examination of the injured area to assist in confirming the diagnosis. Many of these individuals, however, will require the use of an advanced imaging modality such as ultrasound, computed tomography (CT), and/or magnetic resonance imaging (MRI) to increase the accuracy in diagnosing the specific nature of the injury. The purpose of this chapter will be to provide a basic understanding of the four major imaging modalities used in diagnosing injuries: x-ray, ultrasound, CT, and MRI. It will also review pertinent terminology, common imaging applications, and important safety precautions.

 DIAGNOSTIC RADIOGRAPHY

Historical Overview

Using an x-ray tube to produce x-rays and a sheet of x-ray film or image receptor placed in a specially designed cassette to capture the energy of the x-ray beam image is the most commonly used method of taking a radiograph. Since its beginning in the late 1800s, diagnostic radiography, also known as x-ray, has seen several technologic advancements in the design of the x-ray tube, x-ray film, and cassette. Advancements made in image receptor technology have evolved from glass plates, which were used initially, to polyester-base material, which is used currently. Film emulsions have experienced considerable change since they were first introduced. Historically, the x-ray image was produced by the direct exposure of the x-ray beam to the x-ray film. Today, the x-ray image is produced when the x-ray beam interacts with special phosphor crystals within intensifying screens located inside the film cassette. When x-rays interact with the phosphor crystals, a light of a specific wavelength is produced and exposes the x-ray film. This method reduces the amount of radiation necessary to create an x-ray image.

The latest technology incorporates the use of computer technology in what may be referred to as computed radiography or digital radiography. Digital radiography introduces a moving away from the traditional film-screen (hard copy) method of taking an x-ray to producing a digital (soft copy) image that is presented on a high-quality monitor. Digital images, once recorded, can be manipulated just like CT images. The density and contrast scale of the images can be adjusted to demonstrate the anatomy such as bone or soft tissue. The images can be magnified to better visualize small structures. Another advantage of digitally formatted images is that they can be reviewed using high-quality monitors located throughout the hospital in such locations as the emergency room, operating rooms, and patient floors. Soft-copy images can also be sent to other health-care professionals in other health-care settings on a compact disc (CD). Finally, the storage of soft-copy images requires less space than the traditional hard-copy film jacket. The patient's images are stored and maintained on a picture archive and communication system (PACS) for an indefinite period of time.

Radiographic Views

When performing a typical radiographic procedure, the radiologic technologist will position the patient and the anatomic part to be radiographed for two or more radiographic views. These views usually consist of either an anteroposterior (AP) or posteroanterior (PA), an oblique (usually a 45-degree rotation from the AP or PA position) and a lateral (90-degree rotation from AP or PA position). Rotating the anatomy into these angled positions allows the clinician to better define the location of structural change. For some anatomic structures such as wrists, shoulders, and knees, the patient may need to have additional views performed. Additional radiographic views may be required on a patient-by-patient basis. For example, the ulnar flexion may be used to demonstrate a fracture of the navicular bone (Figure 1–1). These various radiographic procedures can be reviewed in radiologic positioning textbooks and manuals (Ballinger and Frank, 2003; Bontrager, 1997; Dowd and Wilson, 1995).

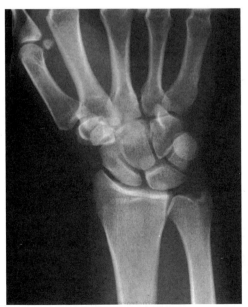 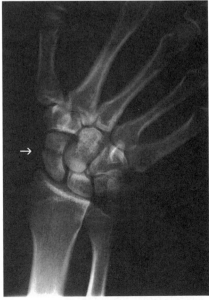

A **B**

Figure 1–1 Posterioranterior (PA) view of the wrist showing the carpal bones. **A.** Routine PA view. **B.** PA view with ulnar deviation. The ulnar deviation position is used specifically to better demonstrate the navicular bone for a possible fracture *(arrow)*.

Advantages and Disadvantages

Diagnostic radiography is the most economic imaging modality. Diagnostic information like fractures, bony lesions (osteoblastic and osteolytic), dislocations, subluxations, and edema may be visible. When soft tissue is imaged for calcification deposits and foreign bodies, it is suggested that the radiographic technique factor kilovoltage (kV) be reduced 10 kV lower than the standard radiographic technique (Dowd and Wilson, 1995). This results in an increase in the subject contrast between soft tissue and bone.

Since diagnostic x-rays produce ionizing radiation, every attempt should be made to protect the patient from the unnecessary exposure that may occur as a result of insufficient patient or examination information, repeat examinations, or performing the wrong examination. To make this process as effective as possible, a qualified physician must complete a request for all radiographic procedures. Pertinent patient information and type of x-ray procedure requested should be provided on the x-ray request form in an accurate and legible manner. Any additional information or concern that may benefit the quality or safety of the x-ray procedure should be communicated (e.g., patient history, patients that may require sedation, pregnancy) to either the radiologic technologist or the radiologist.

ULTRASOUND

Current Status

The applications of ultrasound to the medical field subsequently followed the development of sonar (**so**und **na**vagation **r**anging) and its use during World War II. Since its earlier uses in medical imaging, medical diagnostic sonography, sometimes referred to as sonography or ultrasound, has experienced substantial growth in its applications in imaging the human body. From its initial uses in obstetrics and gynecology to imaging small abdominal structures and assisting with biopsy procedures to its current use in vascular, echocardiographic, and now musculoskeletal imaging, ultrasound continues to make significant contributions to medical imaging (Lin et al., 2000a–d).

The concept of using conventional ultrasound to evaluate the musculoskeletal system is not a new idea. It dates back to the late 1970s (Jacobson, 2002; Jacobson and van Holsbeeck, 1998). The advancements made in ultrasound with the development of high-frequency transducers in the range of 5 to 12 MHz (Jacobson and van Holsbeeck, 1998; Bücklein et al., 2000; Winter et al., 2001) has demonstrated the ability to visualize musculoskeletal structures such as tendons (Figure 1–2), ligaments, articular cartilage, fibrocartilage, peripheral nerves, muscles, and bone. In Table 1–1, the echogenesis of musculoskeletal structures is outlined. Higher frequency transducers produce a better signal-to-noise ratio; however, high-frequency transducers are limited to the depth of tissue they can penetrate. Lower frequency transducers, therefore, are used to image deeper structures such as the hip and posterior knee (Bücklein et al., 2000; Jacobson and van Holsbeeck, 1998). These transducers generate images with a lower signal-to-noise ratio.

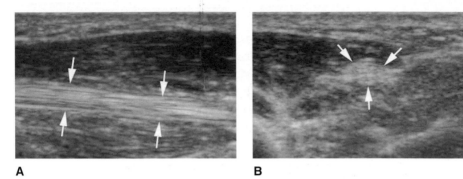

A   **B**

Figure 1–2 Ultrasound image of the of the flexor pollicis longus tendon (arrows). **A.** Longitudinal axis. **B.** Transverse axis.

A new method of imaging called "tissue harmonic imaging," which is different from conventional ultrasound, allows deeper penetration with better image quality compared to conventional ultrasound (Figure 1–3) (Choudhry et al., 2000; Strobel et al., 2004). Conventional ultrasound is accomplished by sending a sound wave from the transducer into a structure and receiving an echo reflected off structures in the body and back to the transducer. In harmonic imaging, instead of listening for the same echo that was sent in the conventional manner, harmonic imaging listens for an echo at twice the transmitted frequency. When harmonic imaging is performed on a patient, the signal coming from the patient does not come from the transducer (transmitted frequency). Instead the echo is generated in the patient as a result of interactions with either tissue or contrast agents. Thus, the echo returning to the transducer travels in only one direction: from the reflective structure to the transducer. This reduction in the distance of travel for the sound beam causes a significant reduction in artifactual noise. The spatial resolution in harmonic imaging is also improved, which permits better visibility of smaller structures.

TABLE 1–1	Echogenesis of Tissue in Ultrasound
Tendons	Longitudinal axis demonstrates a fibrilinear pattern with parallel lines. Transverse axis seen as a round to ovoid shape.
Ligaments	Similar to tendons except with a more compact fibrilinear hyperechoic pattern.
Muscle	Low to midlevel echogenicity with hyperechoic fascial planes.
Nerves	Fascicular structures slightly less echogenic than tendons and ligaments.
Bone cortex	Echogenic surface with posterior acoustic shadowing.
Articular cartilage	Thin hypoechic rim paralleling echogenic articular cortical surface.
Fat	Hyperechoic echotexture sandwiched between skin and muscle layers.

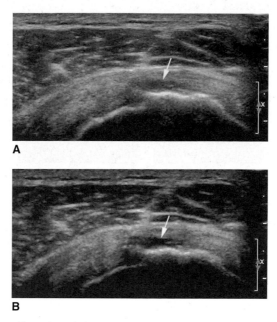

Figure 1–3 Rotator cuff tear *(arrow)* demonstrated. **A.** Conventional ultrasound. **B.** Harmonic imaging.

The high-frequency transducers used with conventional imaging work well for musculoskeletal structures that are near the surface, whereas harmonic imaging allows the use of lower frequency transducers which can penetrate deeper anatomic structures. In studies comparing harmonic imaging to the conventional imaging method in ultrasound, harmonic imaging has demonstrated its superiority over conventional imaging (Choudhry et al., 2000; Strobel et al., 2004).

Advantages and Disadvantages

Ultrasound provides a number of advantages to medical imaging. Ultrasound obtains its image without utilizing harmful ionizing radiation. It is portable, which improves accessibility to the patient and allows for dynamic evaluation of joints. In addition, an ultrasound examination is relatively low in cost compared to other advanced imaging modalities such as CT and MRI (Jacobson, 1999). The use of ultrasound to assist with guided interventional procedures such as aspirations, biopsies, and medication delivery also provides pinpoint accuracy and timely means of diagnosing and treating patients (Sofka and Adler, 2002; Sofka et al., 2001).

Although there are numerous advantages to musculoskeletal ultrasound, operator dependence is probably its best known limitation (Jacobson and van Holsbeeck, 1998). Currently, radiologists interested in applying the benefits of ultrasound to musculoskeletal imaging train sonographers to perform the examination. Radiologists may follow up the examination if there are suspicious areas of concern.

COMPUTED TOMOGRAPHY

Current Status

Computed Tomography has experienced several modifications in its basic design since its initial development in the early 1970s. The most recent technologic advancement, however, was the development of spiral CT (Kalender, 2000; Prokop and Galanski, 2003). Through the development of slip-ring technology used in a spiral CT scanner, the x-ray tube can continuously rotate around the patient as the patient moves through the opening of the CT scanner, whereas conventional CT scanners performed an examination in a slice-by-slice (axial) method. The continuous movement offered through spiral CT greatly reduces scan time, provides volumetric scanning, and multislice capability. The number of slices (images) a CT scanner can acquire per revolution of the x-ray tube depends on the number of rows of detectors. Spiral CT units today may be referred to as multislice or multidetector CT scanners. Over the past few years, the medical profession has experienced a doubling effect in multislice technology. With the current number of slices acquired per revolution in most scanners being 32 slices, some manufactures have already developed and are marketing 64-slice scanners. The future of multislice technology is focused on 128 slices per revolution with a possibility of developing 256-slice units using a different x-ray beam design. These multislice scanners can produce slices that are submillimeter in thickness and can acquire these images in less than a second. Decreasing the slice thickness produces an increase in the spatial resolution and the ability to visualize smaller structures accurately.

Advantages and Disadvantages

Multislice spiral CT (MSCT) provides numerous benefits when imaging the body. With the development of slip-ring technology, the x-ray tube travels around the patient without having to stop and reset itself between slices as was the case with the more conventional CT units. Slip-ring technology allows continuous data acquisition with reduced scan time. Multiple detector channels collect the x-rays as they exit the patient. The number of detectors activated indicates the number of slices and the slice thickness acquired per x-ray tube revolution. In some cases, the CT examination can be performed in a single breath-hold, which helps to eliminate respiratory motion. In performing a chest examination, the chance of missing a lesion along the border of the diaphragm, such as in the lung base or liver, is reduced. Since CT images are in a digital (soft-copy) format, they can be windowed to focus on the soft tissue, lung tissue, or bony tissue by adjusting the density and contrast scale of the image data. This allows the patient to be scanned once with the possibility of viewing the patient's images in a choice of window settings that best depicts the anatomy and pathology. Other benefits offered through the use of MSCT are the high-quality images produced through various software-generated reconstruction methods. These reconstruction methods include multiplanar reformation (MPR) (Prokop and Galanski, 2003), maximum intensity projection (MIP) (Prokop and Galanski, 2003), shaded surface display (SSD), and volume rendering (VR) (Prokop and Galanski, 2003; Pretorius and Fishman, 1999; Ohashi et al., 2004). Multiplanar reformatted images (Figures 1–4 and 1–5) are two-dimensional images that have been

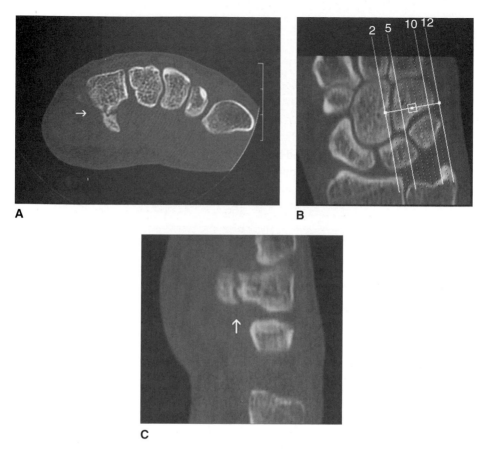

Figure 1–4 CT of the wrist demonstrating a fracture of the hamate. **A.** Axial image showing fracture *(arrow)*. **B.** Coronal MPR image with sagittal slice overlay. **C.** Sagittal MPR image showing fracture *(arrow).*

reconstructed through a computer software process using the previously acquired axial images. MPR images are commonly reformatted into coronal or sagittal images. This reconstruction method is usually used in musculoskeletal and spine (Figure 1–6) applications but may also be used in other areas including the brain, thorax, abdomen, and pelvis. The MIP reconstruction method can be used in vascular applications; however, it is commonly used in MR angiography (MRA). In this reconstruction method, only the voxels with the brightest intensity (maximum intensity) are selected and reconstructed to form the image. Images reconstructed with the SSD (Figure 1–7) method provide a realistic three-dimensional (3D) view of the surface of the structure. Applications for SSD include orthopedic and vascular structures. Volume rendering is a complex, yet versatile, three-dimensional reconstruction method that combines the characteristics of SSD and MIP. Anatomic structures of interest are identified from the initial axial images by their respective CT number, and the VR reconstruction method is applied. Color coding of the tissues may be performed, thus allowing for visual differentiation of various tissues (Figure 1–8). VR is quickly becoming the 3D method of choice due

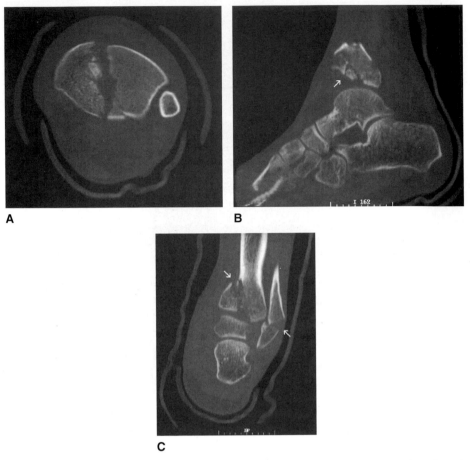

Figure 1–5 Severely comminuted and angulated bimalleolar fracture of the ankle. **A.** Axial CT through lower leg. **B.** Sagittal MPR showing fracture *(arrow)*. **C.** Coronal MPR demonstrating bimalleolar fracture *(arrows)*.

to the speed at which CT workstations are able to process data. Images that are reconstructed using MIP, SSD, or VR can be rotated and viewed from any angle to provide a better understanding of complex 3D structures. Probably the two most common disadvantages associated with CT is the possible risk of an adverse reaction to an intravenous (IV) contrast agent if required and the increased concern regarding the use of CT (particularly in children) as the amount of radiation exposure is significant.

 ## MAGNETIC RESONANCE IMAGING

Current Technology

Since the introduction of MRI in the early 1980s, technologic advancements continue to develop and expand at an ever-increasing pace. Initially used for imaging the brain and spinal cord, MRI use has spread to include numerous applications covering the entire

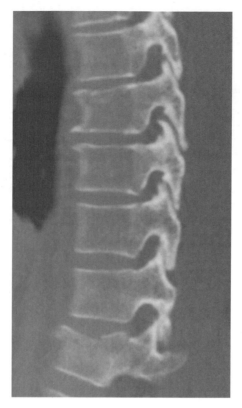

Figure 1–6 Sagittal MPR image showing multiple compression fractures of the thoracic spine.

body. MRI, the most technologically advanced imaging modality to date, can offer a wide range of imaging capabilities through the use of a strong external magnetic field, an arsenal of imaging radiofrequency (RF) coils, a variety of pulse sequences, and the availability of contrast media.

In the area of musculoskeletal imaging (Berquist, 2001; Boutin et al., 2002), MRI has established its presence as a dominating imaging modality useful in diagnosing a wide variety of injuries, disorders, and complications. Once thought of as only being able to be imaged in low- to mid-field strength units, structures involving the musculoskeletal system are increasingly being imaged in high-field units. This again is the result of a variety of technologic advancements incorporated into MRI. Through the use of application-specific (RF) imaging coils, such as surface coils, flexible coils, and coils commonly referred to by the anatomy they have been designed to image such as knee, shoulder, and temporomandibular joint (TMJ), imaging the musculoskeletal system has made significant advancements. The development of pulse sequences and their applications continue to increase and expand.

Overall, there are four basic pulse sequences that have been developed. They include spin echo (SE), gradient echo (GE), inversion recovery (IR), and echo planar imaging (EPI). Using a variety of parameters associated with MRI such as repetition time (TR), echo

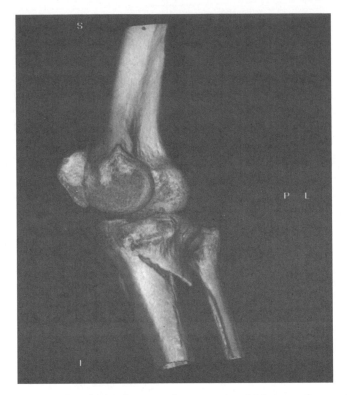

Figure 1–7 Shaded surface display demonstrating a complex tibial plateau fracture involving both medial and lateral aspects of the tibia. Note the SSD image is rotated to show a posterior oblique view of the fracture.

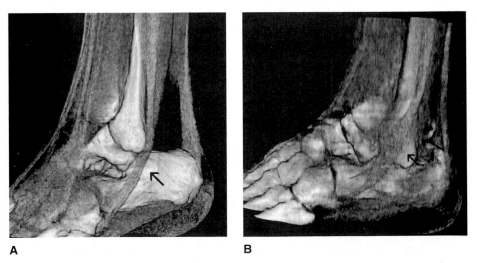

A   B

Figure 1–8 Volume-rendering reconstruction method demonstrating (A) normal peroneus longus tendon *(arrow)* and (B) torn peroneus longus tendon *(arrow)*. (Also see color insert).

time (TE), inversion time (TI), and flip angle (FA), pulse sequences can be adjusted to produce images that provide information that is either T1-weighted, proton density-weighted, T2-weighted, T2*-weighted, or IR. The signal intensity of tissues will vary depending on the imaging parameters used for a given pulse sequence (Table 1–2). Imaging protocols are usually established by the radiologist to provide the most beneficial information to assist with making a diagnosis. Imaging protocols usually are designed to include a combination of pulse sequences obtained in different imaging planes such as transverse (axial), sagittal, coronal, and oblique (orthogonal) to better differentiate between normal and abnormal anatomic structures and to assess trauma in an effort to better diagnose the patient.

An in-depth discussion of these pulse sequences is beyond the scope of this chapter. A brief statement, however, about each pulse sequence should shed light on the information it provides to the overall outcome of the MRI examination. T1-weighted images (Figure 1–9) are best used to demonstrate anatomic detail, whereas T2-weighted images (Figure 1–10) are typically used to identify pathologic conditions. Proton density–weighted images (Figure 1–11) indicate the concentration of hydrogen protons and are beneficial in assessing articular cartilage. Images that are T2*-weighted (Figure 1–12) may exhibit an angiographic, a myelographic, or an arthrographic effect. Inversion recovery pulse sequences such as short-tau IR (STIR) (Figure 1–13) and fluid attenuated IR (FLAIR) are used to null the signal coming from a specific tissue such as fat or cerebrospinal fluid (CSF), respectively. Nulling the signal from a specific tissue allows the surrounding tissue with similar relaxation (signal) characteristics to be visible. A STIR pulse sequence, commonly used in musculoskeletal imaging, is used to null the signal from fat. This allows better visibility of free fluid and partial or complete

TABLE 1–2	Signal Intensity of Tissue in MRI			
Tissue	**T1-weighted**	**Proton density-weighted**	**T2-weighted**	**T2*-weighted**
Cortical bone	Low (dark)	Low (dark)	Low (dark)	Low (dark)
Muscle	Intermediate (moderate)	Intermediate (moderate)	Low (dark)	Low (dark)
Ligament	Low (dark)	Low (dark)	Low (dark)	Low (dark)
Tendon	Low (dark)	Low (dark)	Low (dark)	Low (dark)
Fibrocartilage	Low (dark)	Low (dark)	Low (dark)	Llow (dark)
Articular cartilage	Intermediate (moderate)	Intermediate (moderate)	Low (dark)	High (bright)
Intervertebral disk				
Normal	Low (dark)	Low (dark)	Low (dark)	Low (dark)
Nucleus pulposus	Intermediate (moderate)	Intermediate (moderate)	High (bright)	High (bright)
Degenerative	Low (dark)	Low (dark)	Low (dark)	Low (dark)
Cerebrospinal fluid	Low (dark)	Low (dark)	High (bright)	High (bright)
Fat	High (bright)	High (bright)	Intermediate (moderate)	Low (dark)

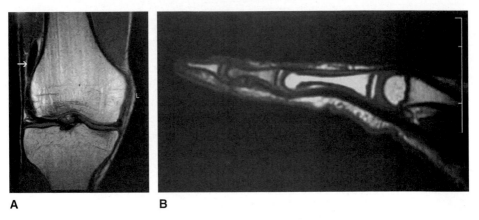

A   **B**

Figure 1–9 T1-weighted images. **A.** Coronal image of the knee demonstrating joint effusion *(arrow)*. **B.** Sagittal image of the index finger demonstrating osteomyelitis of the middle phalanx (low signal).

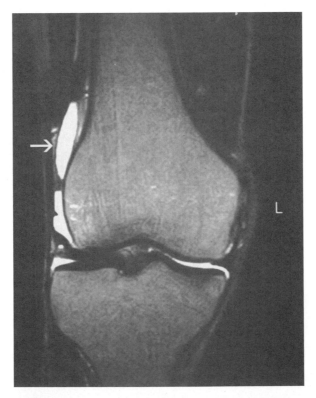

Figure 1–10 T2-weighted fast spin echo coronal of the knee with increased signal characteristic of a tear. Compare with Figure 1–9A.

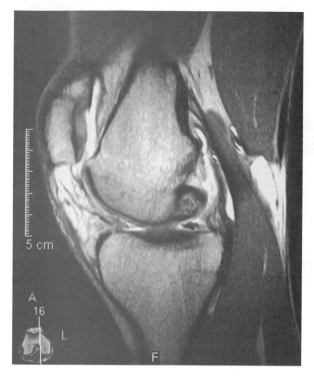

Figure 1–11 Proton density–weighted sagittal image of the knee demonstrating an anterior cruciate ligament tear. Note: Small joint effusion and small popliteal cyst.

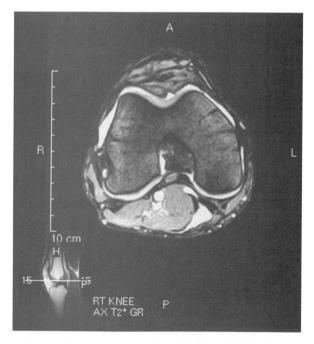

Figure 1–12 T2*-weighted (gradient echo) coronal image of the knee. Note: Small joint effusion and small popliteal cyst.

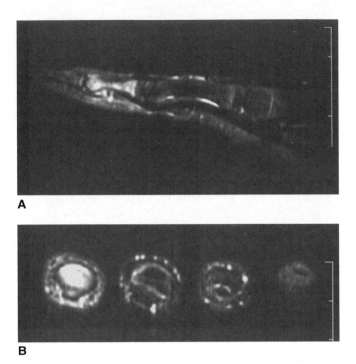

Figure 1–13 STIR pulse sequence demonstrating osteomyelitis (high signal) of the middle phalanx of the index finger. **A.** Sagittal (longitudinal) and **B.** axial views. Compare with Figure 1–9B.

tears. A fat-suppression pulse may also be used to suppress the signal from fat tissue. This may be used in combination with a T2-weighted sequence (Figure 1–14) to better visualize pathology that may be difficult to see because of similar high (bright) signals. When imaging the brain or spinal cord, FLAIR images may be used to null the signal from the CSF, allowing improved visibility of the surrounding periventriclar area of the brain.

MRI is known to produce the best soft tissue contrast of any modality currently available; however, since the development of gadolinium-based MRI contrast agents in 1988, the ability to visualize and identify pathologic conditions has increased. Contrast agents used in MRI are used with a T1-weighted pulse sequence. Historically, these contrast agents were used to assist with the diagnosis of pathologies related to the central nervous system. Since their initial application, however, contrast agents have been used to assess a variety of anatomic structures and assist with demonstrating a variety of other pathologic conditions.

When contrast agents are used in MRI to assess the joint space and surrounding structures, this procedure is commonly referred to as MR arthrography (Berquist, 2001; Steinbach et al., 2002). MR arthrography can be performed using either a direct or indirect technique and can be performed on any joint of the upper or lower extremities. When performing the direct technique for MR arthrography, the patient is initially

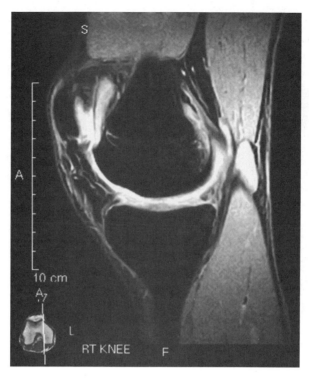

Figure 1–14 T2*-weighted (gradient echo) sagittal image of the knee with fat suppression. Note: Small joint effusion and small popliteal cyst. Compare with Figure 1–11.

brought into the x-ray department and fluoroscopy is used to confirm the intra-articular placement of the needle prior to contrast injection. Following the injection of the contrast agent into the joint capsule, the patient is taken to the MRI unit and positioned for the requested study. When performing this "direct" method for an arthrographic examination in MRI, a saline solution or a dilute concentration of the contrast agent may be supplemented as the contrast agent (Figure 1–15). The "indirect" method of performing an MR arthrography involves an intravenous (IV) injection of the contrast agent and imaging the requested area. This method may be used when the direct approach is either inconvenient or not logistically feasible.

Kinematic MR imaging (KMRI) is a technique that allows MRI technology to assess the function of the joint in order to detect and diagnose various musculoskeletal conditions. More specifically, KMRI allows the joint to be studied through a range of motion, while under stress, or under a loaded condition (weight-bearing) (Shellock and Powers, 2001; Weishaupt and Boxheimer, 2003). Some MRI units are specially designed and may be referred to as "dedicated" or "extremity" MR systems, and incorporate specific positioning devices and RF coils to facilitate the imaging of the joint. Other MR units incorporate devices to simulate weight-bearing conditions. In addition to performing kinematic imaging on the spine, joints such as the hip, knee, ankle, shoulder, wrist, and temporomandibular may also be imaged.

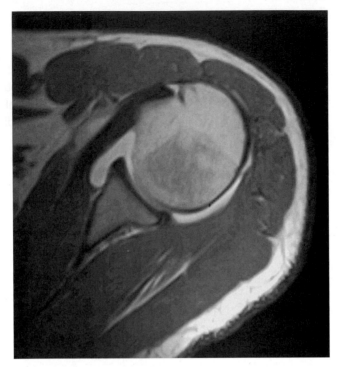

Figure 1–15 T1-weighted axial image of a normal (direct) shoulder arthrogram.

Advantages and Disadvantages

MRI has proven itself to be beneficial to the diagnostic evaluation of the patient and, is in many situations, the gold standard of imaging. The biggest drawbacks would probably be the overall cost of the examination and some contraindications associated with the magnetic field.

The benefits of MRI include excellent soft tissue contrast, increased visibility of tissue without bone artifact, and no ionizing radiation. Since there is no ionizing radiation involved in the procedure, follow-up examinations and imaging of pediatric patients and pregnant patients can be performed safely.

Since the magnetic field of most MRI units is on 24 hours a day, 7 days a week, strict safety guidelines must be followed. The safe utilization of MRI incorporates a screening of all patients and personnel prior to entering into the MR environment to rule out any contraindication that may pose a danger to the individual or health-care personnel.

It is the responsibility of the MRI technologist to conduct the screening of the patient and to decide if there appears to be a contraindication to performing the requested examination. The technologist consults with the radiologist regarding any questionable information presented during the screening of the patient prior to performing the examination. The radiologist will ultimately make the final decision of whether the MRI examination can be performed safely.

Owing to the vast number of biomedical implants, materials, and devices available, the specific contraindications are beyond the scope of this book; however, MRI technologists and radiologists routinely consult the *Reference Manual for Magnetic Resonance Safety, Implants and Devices* (Shellock, 2005) or check online at www.MRIsafety.com for information pertaining to the recommended safety status of a particular product. The safety information provided in the reference manual and listed online requires the technologist to obtain specific information about the type of biomedical implant, material, or device; the name of the manufacturer; and the model number. If the product has been tested in the MRI environment, the results will indicate whether it is safe to perform the MRI examination or if there is a contraindication danger to the patient or the possibility of disabling the function of the implant. It may be required for the patient to provide documentation of the implanted device prior to performing the MRI examination.

 ## TERMS

Ultrasound

Echogenic: Describes a structure that produces echoes.
Hyperechoic: An increase in echoes (more echogenic) within a structure.
Hypoechoic: A decrease in echoes (less echogenic) within a structure.
Isoechoic: Describes two structures having the same acoustic echogenicity.
Anechoic: Without echoes.

Computed Tomography

Multislice/multidetector CT: A CT scanner capable of acquiring more than one slice simultaneously per revolution of the x-ray tube. The number of slices acquired is dependent on the number of detector rows.
Spiral CT: A method of scanning with continuous rotation of the x-ray tube and simultaneous continuous translation of the patient in the z-direction.
Windowing: The process of adjusting the window center (density) and window width (contrast) of the displayed image.

Magnetic Resonance Imaging

Repetition time (TR): The time between the beginning of one excitation pulse in a pulse sequence to the next excitation pulse in the same pulse sequence.
Echo time (TE): The between the mid point of the excitation pulse and the rephasing of the protons.
Inversion time (TI): The time between the initial 180-degree RF pulse and the subsequent 90-degree excitation pulse. Used in IR pulse sequences such as STIR and FLAIR.
Flip angle (FA): Refers to the angle of rotation of the net magnetization vector (NMV or M) produced by an RF pulse. Flip angles are measured relative from the longitudinal (z) axis of the main magnetic field (βo). For example, a 90-degree FA rotates the NMV from the longitudinal plane (Mz) into the transverse plane (Mxy).

T1-weighted: A pulse sequence using a short TR and short TE value to demonstrate the differences of tissues T1 relaxation. This sequence is commonly used to demonstrate the anatomy.

Proton (Spin) density—weighted: A pulse sequence using a long TR and short TE value to demonstrate the concentration of hydrogen protons; the higher the concentration of hydrogen protons, the higher (brighter) the signal.

T2-weighted: A spin echo pulse sequence using a long TR and long TE value to demonstrate the differences between tissues with different T2 (spin-spin) relaxation times. This sequence is commonly used to identify pathology.

T2*-weighted (T-two-star): The gradient echo version of a T2-weighted spin echo pulse sequence. This pulse sequence is faster than a spin echo pulse sequence. T2* images are composed of spin-spin relaxation and inhomogeneities of the magnetic field. Image contrast in gradient echo pulse sequence depends on T2*.

Inversion recovery: A pulse sequence such as STIR or FLAIR that consists of an initial 180-degree pulse to invert the net magnetization followed by 90-degree and 180-degree pulses to generate a spin echo signal.

Spin echo: A pulse sequence consisting of a 90-degree excitation pulse followed by a 180-degree rephasing pulse.

Gradient echo: A pulse sequence consisting of a FA (≤90-degree) excitation pulse and a gradient reversal.

 ## REFERENCES

Ballinger, P. W., & Frank, E. D. (2003). *Merrill's atlas of radiographic positions and Radiologic procedures.* 10th ed. Vols. 1–3. St. Louis: Mosby.

Berquist, T. H. (Ed.). (2001). *MRI of the musculoskeletal system.* 4th ed. New York: Lippincott Williams & Wilkins.

Bontrager, K. L. (1997). *Textbook of radiographic positioning and related anatomy.* 4th ed. St. Louis: Mosby.

Boutin, R. D., Fritz, R. C., & Steinbach, L. S. (2002). Imaging of sports-related muscle injuries. *Radiologic Clinics of North America, 37*(40), 333–362.

Bücklein, W., Vollert, K., Wohlgemuth, W. A., & Bohndorf, K. (2000). Ultrasonography of acute musculoskeletal disease. *European Radiology, 10*(2), 290–296.

Choudhry, S., Gorman, B., Charboneau, J. W., Tradup, D. J., Beck, R. J., Kofler, J. M., et al. (2000). Comparison of tissue harmonic imaging with conventional US in abdominal disease. *Radiographics, 20,* 1127–1135.

Dowd, S. B., & Wilson, B. G. (1995). *Encyclopedia of radiographic positioning.* Vols. 1 & 2 — It is a two volume set 1–2. Philadelphia: Saunders.

Jacobson, J. A. (1999). Musculoskeletal sonography and MR imaging: A role for both imaging methods. *Radiologic Clinics of North America, 37*(4), 713–735

Jacobson, J. A. (2002). Ultrasound in sports medicine. *Radiologic Clinics of North America, 40,* 363–386.

Jacobson, J. A., & van Holsbeeck, M. T. (1998). Musculoskeletal ultrasound. *Orthopedic Clinics of North America, 29*(1), 135–167.

Kalender, W. A. (2000). *Computed tomography: Fundamental, system technology, image quality, applications*. Munich: Publicis MCD Verlag.

Lin, J., Fessell, D. P., Jacobson, J. A., Weadock, W. J., & Hayes, C. W. (2000a). An illustrated tutorial of musculoskeletal sonography: Part 1, introduction and general principles [Electronic version]. *American Journal of Roentgenology, 175*, 637–645.

Lin, J., Jacobson, J. A., Fessell, D. P., Weadock, W. J., & Hayes, C. W. (2000b). An illustrated tutorial of musculoskeletal sonography: Part 2, upper extremity [Electronic version]. *American Journal of Roentgenology, 175*, 1071–1079.

Lin, J., Fessell, D. P., Jacobson, J. A., Weadock, W. J., & Hayes, C. W. (2000c). An illustrated tutorial of musculoskeletal sonography: Part 3, lower extremity. [Electronic version]. *American Journal of Roentgenology, 175*, 1313–1321.

Lin, J., Jacobson, J. A., Fessell, D. P., Weadock, W. J., & Hayes, C. W. (2000d). An illustrated tutorial of musculoskeletal sonography: Part 4, musculoskeletal masses, sonographically guided interventions, and miscellaneous topics. [Electronic version]. *American Journal of Roentgenology, 175*, 1711–1719.

Ohashi, K., El-Khoury, G. Y., & Bennett, D. L. (2004). MDCT of tendon abnormalities using volume-rendering images. *American Journal of Roentgenology, 182*, 161–165.

Pretorius, E. S., & Fishman, E. K. (1999). Volume-rendering three dimensional spiral CT: Musculoskeletal applications. *Radiographics, 19*, 1143–1160.

Prokop, M., & Galanski, M. (2003). *Spiral and multislice computed tomography of the body*. New York: Thieme.

Shellock, F. G. (2005). *Reference manual for magnetic resonance safety, implants and devices: 2005 edition*. Los Angles: Biomedical Research Publishing Group.

Shellock, F. G., & Powers, C. M. (Eds.). (2001). *Kinematic MRI of the joints: Functional anatomy, kinesiology, and clinical applications*. Boca Raton, FL: CRC Press.

Sofka, C. M., & Adler, R. S. (2002). Ultrasound-guided interventions in the foot and ankle. *Seminars in Musculoskeletal Radiology, 6*(2), 163–168.

Sofka, C. M., Collins, A. J., & Adler, R. S. (2001). Use of ultrasonographic guidance in interventional musculoskeletal procedures: A review from a single institution. *Journal of Ultrasound in Medicine, 20*(1), 21–26.

Steinbach, L. S., Palmer, W. E., & Schweitzer, M. E. (2002). Special focus session: MR arthrography [Electronic version]. *Radiographics, 22*, 1223–1246.

Strobel, K., Zanetti, M., Nagy, L., & Hodler, J. (2004). Suspected rotator cuff lesions: Tissue harmonic imaging versus conventional US of the shoulder. *Radiology 230*, 243–249.

Weishaupt, D., & Boxheimer, L. (2003). Magnetic resonance imaging of the weight-bearing spine. *Seminars in Musculoskeletal Radiology, 7*(4), 277–286.

Winter, T. C., III, Teefey, S. A., & Middleton, W. D. (2001). Musculoskeletal ultrasound: An update. *Radiologic Clinics of North America, 39*(3), 465–483.

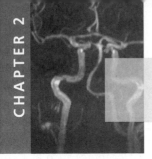

CHAPTER 2

Imaging of the Brain

Computed tomography (CT) and magnetic resonance imaging (MRI) were initially introduced to the medical imaging field in the early 1970s and 1980s, respectively. With their initial application in neuroimaging, their contribution to medical imaging has been tremendous. Subsequent to these beginnings in CT and MRI, numerous imaging applications have been developed to study anatomic structures better, diagnose diseases and disorders of the body systems, and follow treatment patterns. In this chapter, the primary focus will be to provide information on the use of these imaging modalities in neuroimaging as it applies specifically to CT and MRI. An overview, however, of other imaging modalities used in evaluating the brain requires a brief discussion.

Although CT and MRI have taken the spotlight in neuroimaging, basic skull radiography, ultrasound (US), positron emission tomography (PET), and single-emission computed tomography (SPECT) also have their respective roles in assisting the physician in caring for the patient. These imaging modalities can be grouped into two categories according to the type of image information demonstrated. For conventional CT, MRI, and US, images present the morphology of the anatomy within the imaging field-of-view. With PET, SPECT, and the advanced technologies associated with CT, MRI, and US, functional images demonstrate the flow and distribution of blood throughout the brain. Most imaging facilities have the conventional imaging modalities mentioned above available for their physicians' utilization. The advanced imaging technologies that provide functional (physiologic) information are not routinely available in all imaging facilities. For the majority of applications, conventional imaging modalities are sufficient. However, in difficult cases, the functional modalities may be used to assist in detecting diseases and disorders in an earlier stage of development compared to conventional modalities.

Since the development of radiology in 1895, skull radiographs have been used to evaluate patients with head trauma. Skull radiographs taken from several different views may demonstrate fractures and assist with identifying displacement of internal midline structures, which could indicate an intracranial space-occupying mass such as a hematoma. Historically, other radiologic procedures such as pneumoencephalography and cerebral angiography were developed to further the diagnostic ability of radiology in evaluating head trauma. Since the development of CT, pneumoencephalography is no longer used. For trauma patients with a history of mild head injury, a basic x-ray skull series might be ordered as a screening for possible fractures. In some cases, however, where a skull fracture is suspected, a CT of the head is mandatory. Cerebral angiography, a radiologic (x-ray) procedure that is performed to evaluate the blood vessels of the brain is used to examine intracranial vascular lesions such as aneurysms (Figure 2–1), arteriovenous malformations (AVMs), tumors, and atherosclerotic or stenotic lesions. Comparatively, cerebral angiography, still considered to be the "gold standard" when evaluating the cerebral vasculature structures, provides higher spatial resolution than either magnetic resonance angiography (MRA) or computed tomography angiography (CTA). For initial screening examinations, however, imaging procedures such as CTA, MRA, and duplex US have replaced cerebral angiography.

The use of US would not typically be considered for emergency applications. US does have a considerable number of beneficial factors associated with its real-time imaging capability, affordability, portability, and utilization of nonionizing radiation. The ability of US in vascular imaging to provide a method of baseline screening of the carotid arteries and other pertinent vascular structures, to measure blood flow, and to allow safe follow-up examinations is very advantageous. US may be used in neurosurgery to assist in providing anatomic information during intraoperative procedures such as tumor removal, placement of catheters in the ventricles of the brain, and in decompressing and debriding open head injuries. US, as well as CT and MRI, may be useful in performing aspiration and biopsy procedures.

PET uses short-lived radioactive isotopes (radiotracers) injected into a patient to demonstrate various aspects of brain hemodynamics (e.g., cerebral blood flow and cerebral blood volume) and functional information (e.g., metabolic activity). PET imaging is

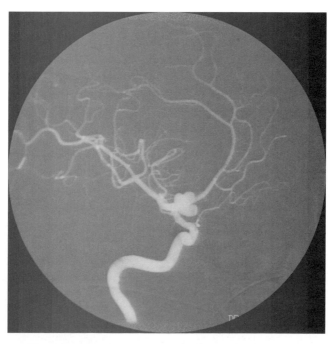

Figure 2–1 An oblique view of the right carotid arteriogram showing a large aneurysm of the right internal carotid artery at its bifurcation.

based on an assumption that areas of high radioactivity are associated with brain activity. The specific radiotracer is chosen based on its similarity to the naturally occurring bio-chemical component of the human body being imaged. The radiotracer emits a positron from its nucleus. After traveling a short distance, the positron collides with an electron in a neighboring atom, producing an annihilation reaction. Two gamma rays (511 keV) are produced and are emitted 180 degrees in opposite directions from the annihilation point. The two gamma rays are then captured by a detector and used to reconstruct a cross-sectional image of the anatomy being imaged. Although PET has demonstrated numerous applications throughout the body, its application in imaging of the brain has been to diagnose tumors, strokes, epilepsy, Alzheimer's disease, Parkinson's disease, Huntington's disease, and various psychiatry disorders. PET may be useful in predicting neurologic outcome of a patient who has experienced traumatic brain injuries.

SPECT is an imaging modality that uses radiotracers to assess stroke patients. Initially developed in the early 1980s, SPECT was used to evaluate the regional cerebral blood flow (rCBF) in patients with acute ischemic strokes. Compared to PET, SPECT provided a less expensive method of neuroimaging. PET, however, is more accurate in measuring the rCBF. Furthermore, with the recent advancements made in CT, patients who histor-ically would have had a SPECT study of the brain are now being studied by CT.

Current state of the art multislice CT units can acquire 64 slices per x-ray tube rota-tion (i.e., 64-slice spiral CT units). The development of 256-slice CT units is in progress and will probably become available in the coming years. These technological advance-ments will no doubt have an impact on improving vascular imaging. With the speed and resolution of multislice CT, it is easy to see why it has become the standard modal-ity to use in the emergency environment, especially in trauma-related situations. There is increasing concern regarding the use of CT (particularly in children) as the amount of radiation exposure is significant.

Like CT, MRI has made considerable technologic advancements. Improvements in magnetic field strength, gradient coils, and faster pulse sequences are a few of the major advancements in MRI. Such technologic advancements include magnetic resonance angiography (MRA), MR perfusion, MR diffusion, MR spectroscopy (MRS), and func-tional MRI (fMRI). An overview of advantages and disadvantages of CT and MRI as they apply to head imaging are provided in Table 2–1.

The assessment of blood vessels can be performed with either conventional CT or MRI. CTA and MRA procedures can be obtained in either a two-dimensional or three-dimensional acquisition and are useful in evaluating the vasculature of the head and neck. These procedures may be used for screening and early detection in an attempt to prevent strokes. A CTA procedure of either the brain (circle of Willis) or neck (carotid arteries) requires an intravenous injection of an iodinated nonionic contrast agent in conjunction with thin-section imaging to demonstrate the morphology of the blood vessels such as stenoses and intracranial aneurysms. An MRA procedure of the brain or neck currently requires one of the two techniques available for a specific examination. Time-of-flight MRA (TOF-MRA) incorporates the use of saturation pulses to reduce the signal in the selected area of interest. The blood entering into the selected area has not

COLOR PLATE

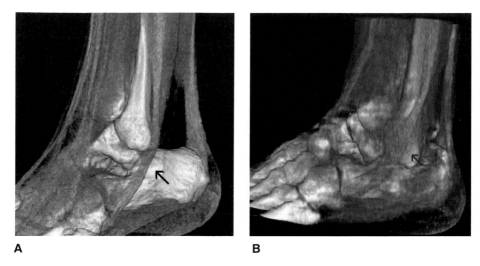

A   **B**

Figure 1–8 Volume-rendering reconstruction method demonstrating (A) normal peroneus longus tendon *(arrow)* and (B) torn peroneus longus tendon *(arrow)*.

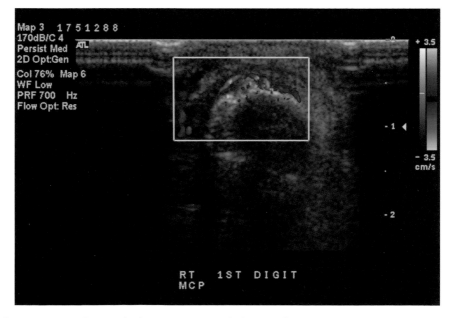

Figure 7–37 A color Doppler image suggesting thickening of the joint capsule with synovial proliferation at the first metacarpophalangeal joint.

TABLE 2–1   Imaging in Head Trauma—Advantages and Disadvantages

Computed Tomography	Magnetic Resonance Imaging
Advantages	*Advantages*
Accessible in emergency facilities	No ionizing radiation
Fast scan time	Noninvasive
Good image detail	Superior contrast resolution
Noninvasive	Orthogonal imaging
Good localization of lesions, foreign bodies, and bony fragments	MR angiography
Multiplanar reformations	Functional studies
CT angiography	
Disadvantages	*Disadvantages*
Ionizing radiation	Contraindications
Artifacts	Scan time
Some skull fractures may be missed	Motion artifacts
	Less accessible in emergency facilities
	Difficult to evaluate bony fractures

CT, computed tomography; MR, magnetic resonance.

been saturated and will produce a relatively large signal. For an MRA procedure of the brain (circle of Willis), the method most commonly used is time-of-flight (Figure 2–2).

The contrast enhanced-MRA (CE-MRA) technique requires an intravenous injection of a T1-weighted paramagnetic (e.g., gadolinium) contrast agent. Although not typically used in imaging the intracranial vessels, CE-MRA is clinically acceptable for imaging the carotid arteries (Figure 2–3). Furthermore, as with any contrast agent injected into a patient, there are specific indications and contraindications that must be observed.

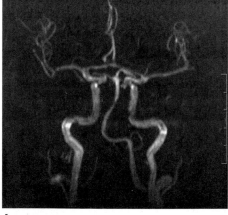
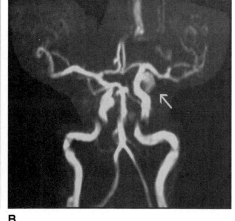

A   **B**

Figure 2–2 Time-of-flight images. **A.** The circle of Willis in an anterior view. **B.** Circle of Willis in an anterior view showing an aneurysm (*arrow*).

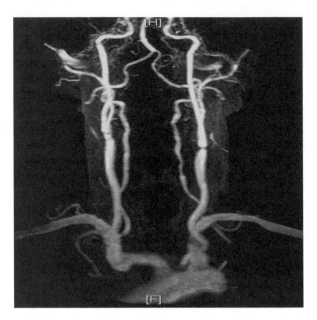

Figure 2–3 Contrast-enhanced MRA (CE-MRA) of the carotid arteries demonstrating a stenosis in the left carotid artery.

Perfusion-based imaging is used to measure the flow of blood through the capillary bed of an organ or tissue region in vivo. Perfusion parameters such as cerebral blood flow (CBF), cerebral blood volume (CBV), and the mean transit time (MTT) are calculated to provide quantitative data. Several different imaging modalities such as CT, MRI, PET, US, SPECT, xenon-enhanced CT may be used to provide perfusion-based images.

CT perfusion used in conjunction with CTA provides complementary information in patient assessment. CT perfusion incorporates a bolus IV injection of a contrast agent into a peripheral vein. Dynamic scanning of the intracranial vessels is performed as the contrast agent washing and washout (first pass) of the area of interest. This produces a series of images covering a section of the brain that demonstrates the distribution of the contrast agent in the brain.

With MRI perfusion imaging, there are two methods that can be performed: dynamic susceptibility contrast (DSC) and arterial spin labeling (ASL). In the dynamic susceptibility contrast approach (DSC-MRI), a paramagnetic contrast agent (gadolinium) is injected to provide information about the perfusion parameters mentioned above. Arterial spin labeling (ASL), which does not use a contrast agent, incorporates radiofrequency (RF) pulses to label moving spins magnetically in flowing blood.

 DIFFUSION-WEIGHTED IMAGING

Diffusion-weighted imaging (DWI) is an MRI technique used to image the translational movement (Brownian motion) of water and other molecules along random paths as they collide with and move past each other. One of the most important pulse sequences developed in several years, DWI has been shown to assist in the detection of ischemic areas of the brain (see Figure 2–10D). Additional applications have been used to differentiate cysts from solid tumors, assist with the diagnosis of inflammatory disorders, and assess white matter abnormalities such as multiple sclerosis (MS). With DWI, areas with reduced diffusion will display a hyperintense (bright) signal.

MAGNETIC RESONANCE SPECTROSCOPY

Magnetic resonance spectroscopy (MRS) is a technique that is used to obtain spectral information in the forms of spectral peaks. Information regarding the nuclei being analyzed during the MRS examination is based on the frequency or chemical shift, peak amplitude, and the area under the peak of the nuclei. Although there are several nuclei that can be evaluated with MRS, ^{1}H proton is specifically used for neurologic applications. Clinical applications for neurologic MRS have been used to assist with the evaluation of brain tumors, AIDS patients, stroke and ischemia, Alzheimer's disease, head trauma, and Gulf War syndrome.

FUNCTIONAL MRI

Functional MR imaging (fMRI) of the brain is used to assist in identifying different areas of brain activity as a result of increased blood flow to the activated cortex. This is accomplished by using a technique commonly referred to as BOLD (blood oxygenation level dependent) to detect changes in blood flow. Images are acquired during a paradigm that consists of a series alternating between a specific activity or stimulus and a rest phase and a variety of brain areas (motor, sensory, visual, etc) have been mapped. The metabolic activity of neurons can be measured with this technique. This can also be beneficial in presurgical planning to map vital areas such as motor, language, and memory. Knowing the location and distance between important structures of the cortex and a lesion is significant in reducing the risk of a postoperative deficit.

Less expensive than CTA and MRA, Doppler US provides a method to measure the cerebral blood flow in patients that is more affordable and can be conveniently performed at the patient's bedside. Doppler US is performed without the use of ionizing radiation and can be repeated as often as clinically indicated. While some information on blood flow can be acquired from the large extracranial vessels (internal carotid artery) in the neck region, little information regarding areas of specific perfusion is furnished.

Xenon-enhanced computed tomography (XeCT) utilizes a CT scanner and a xenon inhalation delivery system. The xenon gas used is stable, is not radioactive, and serves as a contrast agent to assess the cerebral blood flow. Initial CT images are acquired without xenon gas and are used as a baseline scan. Specific slice levels are then selected and used to evaluate the patient's CBF during the inhalation of xenon gas. The patient then inhales a mixture of xenon and oxygen for a prescribed period of time during which the CT scanner acquires several images of each of the previous selected slice levels. Following the study, the normal cerebral tissue will appear enhanced while abnormal areas have reduced enhancement. The Food and Drug Administration (FDA) has not approved XeCT use in the United States.

TRAUMATIC BRAIN INJURY

According to the Centers for Disease Control and Prevention's (CDC) *Injury Fact Book*, approximately 1.4 million Americans sustain a traumatic brain injury (TBI) annually. Further, Thurman, et al., 1999 (as cited in the National Center of Injury Prevention and Control, 2007), estimated that roughly 5.3 million Americans—2 percent of the US population—currently live with disabilities resulting from TBI. From a financial viewpoint, Finkelstein Corso, Miller and Associates (as cited in the National Center for Injury Prevention and Control, 2007) estimated the direct medical costs and indirect costs such as lost productivity of TBI at $60 billion in the United States in 2000. The Brain Injury Association of America (1986) states,

> *Traumatic brain injury is an insult to the brain, not of a degenerative or congenital nature but caused by an external physical force, that may produce a diminished or altered state of consciousness, which results in an impairment of cognitive abilities or physical functioning.*

Further, in an effort to compare TBI to other leading injuries and diseases, TBIs are approximately 8 times higher than new cases of breast cancer and 34 times higher than HIV/AIDS. Traumatic brain injuries that will be discussed include epidural hematomas, subdural hematomas, and subarachnoid hemorrhages (SAHS).

Epidural Hematoma

An epidural hematoma (EDH) is a traumatic accumulation of blood that is located between the inner table of the skull and the dura mater (Figure 2–4). Often the result

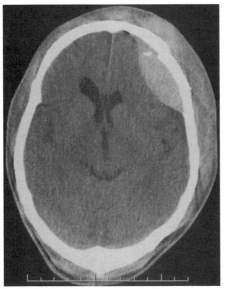

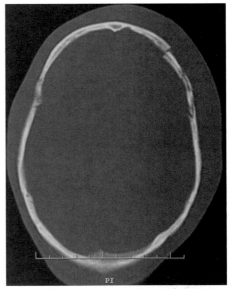

A   **B**

Figure 2–4 Epidural hematoma. **A.** Noncontrast CT shows a typical biconvex hyperdense acute left frontal epidural hematoma with mass effect on the left frontal lobe. **B.** Bone window setting demonstrating a left frontal skull fracture.

of a blunt force to the head, the majority (80 percent or higher) of EDHs occur in the temporoparietal region of the skull. While approximately 90 percent of EDHs involve the meningeal arteries, 10 percent may result in tearing the dural sinuses and veins that course through the impacted area. Fractures occurring in the temporoparietal region usually cause a tearing of the middle meningeal artery. Epidural hematomas may also be located in the frontal (10 percent) and occipital (10 percent) regions of the skull. An EDH would characteristically appear biconvex on either CT or MRI examinations. The biconvex shape occurs as a result of the outer border following the inner table of the skull and the inner border being limited by the dural attachment to the skull.

On CT, traumatic brain injuries are usually evaluated with two computer-generated window settings: (1) brain window setting and (2) bone window setting. The brain window setting is useful in evaluating the anatomic structures of the brain to see if there is any evidence of pneumocephalus, hydrocephalus, cerebral edema, midline shift, or compression of the ventricular system of the brain. In the brain window setting, an epidural hematoma will appear with the characteristic biconvex-shaped hematoma. In the acute stage, the hematoma will appear bright or hyperdense. In the subacute stage, the hematoma will appear isodense to surrounding brain tissue. In the chronic stage, the hematoma will appear dark or hypodense. The bone window setting is useful to visualize bony factures of the skull and facial area, as well as bony fragments that may be scattered within the impacted area. In Table 2–2, an overview of the imaging characteristics for an epidural hematoma, subdural hematoma (SDH), and SAH is provided.

Subdural Hematoma

A SDH is a collection of blood located in the subdural space between the dura mater and the arachnoid mater (Figures 2–5 and 2–6). On CT and MRI, the characteristic appearance of a SDH is crescent with possible mass effect. Subdural hematomas tend to occur more commonly in elderly people as a result of blunt trauma to the head such as a fall, but are seldom associated with a skull fracture. In elderly patients, the combined effects of cerebral atrophy along with less resilient cerebral veins allows for an increase in brain motion which tear the cerebral veins. In young patients, the most common method of injury is a motor vehicle accident when a high-velocity deceleration action tears cerebral veins. In mild to moderate closed head injuries, up to 30 percent of patients may experience a SDH. Acute SDHs may be divided into two groups, simple or complicated, depending on parenchymal brain tissue involvement. A simple SDH implies there is no

TABLE 2–2	Imaging Characteristics of Hematoma			
Stage	**Time Period**	**T1-Weighted**	**T2-Weighted**	**CT**
Hyperacute	<24 hours	Slightly hypointense	Slightly Hyperintense	
Acute	1–3 days	Slightly hypointense	Hypointense	Hyperdense
Subacute				Isodense
Early	4–7 days	Hyperintense	Hypointense	
Late	1–2 weeks	Hyperintense	Hyperintense	
Chronic	>2 weeks	Hypointense	Hypointense	Hypodense

CT, computed tomography.

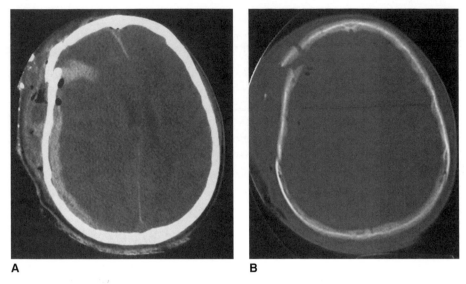

A   **B**

Figure 2–5 Subdural hematoma. **A.** Noncontrast CT showing a crescentic high-density acute right subdural hematoma in the right parietal and occipital region with mass effect on the right lateral ventricle and midline shift to the left. There is also a right frontal lobe intracerebral hematoma as well as pneumocephalus. **B.** Bone windowing setting shows a skull fracture of the right frontal bone.

parenchymal injury present. Approximately half of all SDHs are simple; the remaining are considered to be complicated with parenchymal injury. A mortality rate of approximately 20 percent is associated with simple SDHs, whereas there is a mortality rate of about 50 percent associated with complicated SDHs.

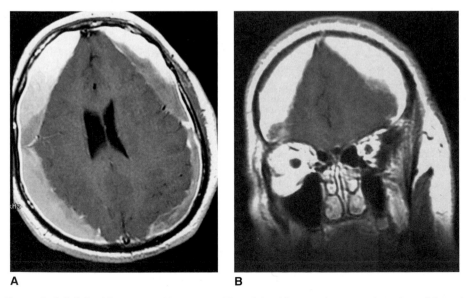

A   **B**

Figure 2–6 Subdural hematoma. Noncontrast T1-weighted images demonstrating a large bilateral subdural hematoma (high signal). **A.** Axial. **B.** Coronal.

Subarachnoid Hemorrhage

A subarachnoid hemorrhage (SAH) implies a collection of blood within the subarachnoid space located between the arachnoid mater and the pia mater (Figure 2–7). Although SAHs may result because of a traumatic event, they may also be categorized as nontraumatic. The scope of this section will focus on nontraumatic SAHs. Nontraumatic SAHs occur most often as a result of a ruptured saccular (berry) aneurysm (Figures 2–1 and 2–8). Other causes may include intracranial arteriovenous malformations (AVMs) (Figure 2–9) or hypertension. The number of SAHs vary from 6 to 25 cases per 100,000 individuals per year. A noncontrast CT examination is the modality of choice for the diagnosis of a subarachnoid hemorrhage and demonstrates blood in the subarachnoid space (e.g., basilar cisterns and sylvian fissures) of the brain. CTA studies in conjunction with 3D-postprocessing technique may reveal an aneurysm. Likewise, conventional MRI and MRA procedures may demonstrate an intracranial aneurysm; however, T1- and T2-weighted images may not be helpful in showing a SAH. The fluid-attenuated inversion recovery (FLAIR) pulse sequence is useful and very sensitive in showing blood (hyperintense) in the subarachnoid space. The majority (80 percent) of these cases are related to intracranial aneurysms. Complaints of severe headaches, loss of consciousness, and focal neurologic deficits are signs and symptoms associated with a SAH.

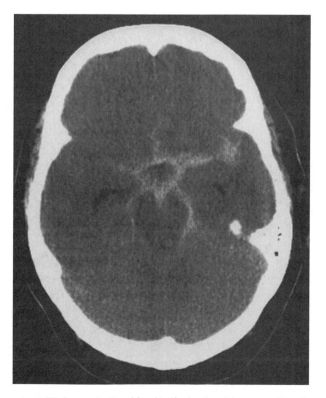

Figure 2–7 Noncontrast CT demonstrating blood in the basilar cisterns as will as the sylvian fissures.

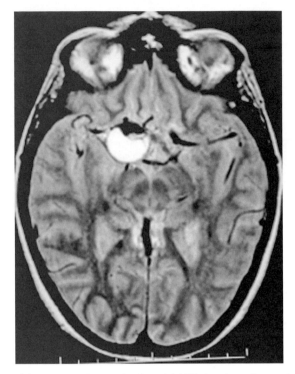

Figure 2–8 Intracranial aneurysm. Proton-density axial MRI showing a large mixed signal intensity aneurysm of the right internal carotid artery.

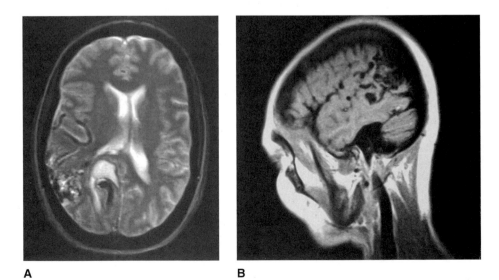

A   B

Figure 2–9 Arteriovenous malformation. MR images demonstrate a collection of signal void worms in the right posterior parietal and occipital lobes. **A.** T2-weighted axial. **B.** T1-weighted sagittal.

CEREBROVASCULAR ACCIDENTS

Cerebrovascular accidents (CVAs), or strokes, can be classified as either ischemic (Figure 2–10) or hemorrhagic (Figure 2–11). Depending on the type of stroke, patients may appear with a sudden onset of focal neurologic deficits, varying degree of paralysis, visual field

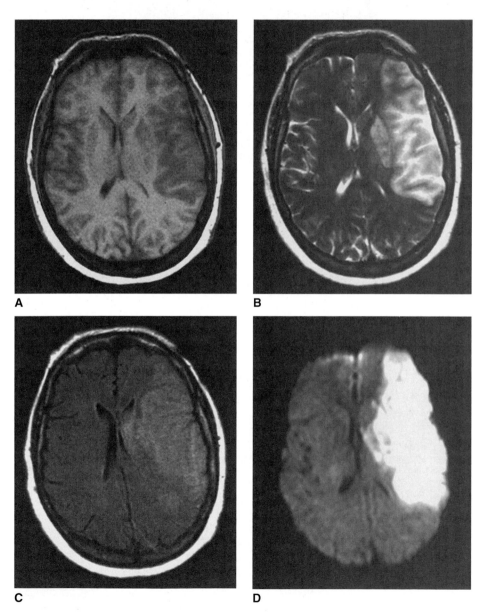

A

B

C

D

Figure 2–10 Ischemic stroke. Large acute left middle cerebral arterial infarct. **A.** T1-weighted. **B.** T2-weighted. **C.** Fluid-attenuated inversion recovery (FLAIR). **D.** Diffusion-weighted image (DWI).

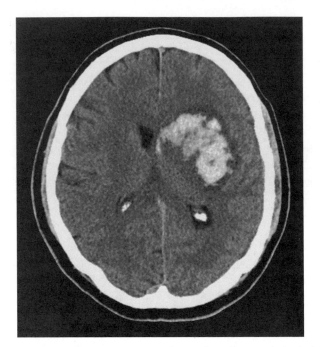

Figure 2–11 Hemorrhagic stroke. Noncontrast CT shows a large hematoma in the left basal ganglia with some surrounding edema. There is compression of the left lateral ventricle and some midline shift to the right. Note: Calcified choroid plexus in the lateral ventricles bilaterally.

deficits, ataxia, vertigo, aphasia, or loss of consciousness. Currently, strokes affect approximately 750,000 people a year; however, it is estimated that as the Baby Boomers continue to age, the number of strokes annually will increase. The majority, 85 percent, of all CVAs are ischemic, and occur secondary to artherothrombosis and cardioembolism. The remaining 15 percent of strokes are hemorrhagic and result from such factors as hypertension, ruptured intracranial aneurysm, anticoagulant therapy, thrombolytic therapy, drug abuse, AVMs, asculitis, intracranial neoplasms, and history of prior stroke.

 DEMYELINATING DISEASE

Multiple Sclerosis

MS is an inflammatory demyelinating disease affecting the white matter tracts of the central nervous system (Figure 2–12). This progressive disease is further characterized by the destruction of the myelin sheath that insulates the axon part of the nerve cell. The areas of demyelination are commonly referred to as *plaques*. MS may go through periods of exacerbation and remission.

The occurrence of MS varies depending on both the ethnic background and geographic environment. MS is most commonly seen in white people of northern European descent and those living in climates that are neither very hot nor very cold. Approximately

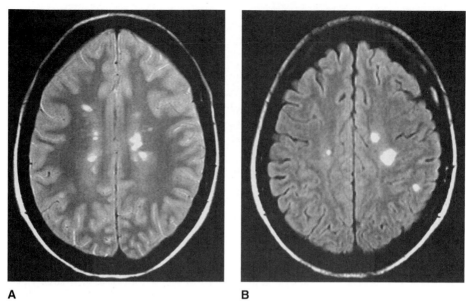

A   **B**

Figure 2–12 Multiple sclerosis. **A.** MR proton-density axial image shows ovoid hyperintense lesions in the centrum semiovale bilaterally. **B.** Postcontrast T1-weighted axial shows enhancement of active multiple sclerosis plaques.

1 in every 1000 people is affected. Females are slightly more affected than males with a 3 to 2 ratio. MS usually occurs between the ages of 18 and 50 years; however, MS can affect any age group.

Prior to MRI, CT was used to rule out other causes for the neurologic impairments, but was unable to demonstrate a diagnostic value in detecting MS. The use of CT in conjunction with IV contrast media attempted to identify active MS plaques but failed. CT can be used to assess the degree of cerebral atrophy associated with MS.

The introduction of MRI in medical imaging has changed the course of diagnosing and monitoring MS. Through the use of a variety of pulse sequences, MRI is able to demonstrate MS plaques clearly without the use of ionizing radiation. With the use of an IV contrast media and T1-weighted imaging, active MS plaques may be enhanced. In Table 2–3, an overview of imaging characteristics for MS is provided.

TABLE 2–3	MRI Imaging Characteristics for Multiple Sclerosis
T1-weighted images	Plaques appear isointense to hypointense
Proton density-weighted images	Plaques appear hyperintense
T2-weighted images	Plaques appear hyperintense
FLAIR images	Plaques appear hyperintense
T1-weighted images with IV contrast	Active plaques may appear hyperintense

NEURODEGERATIVE DISORDERS

Dementia is a broad term used to characterize a general loss of intellectual abilities involving impairment of memory, judgment, and abstract thinking as well as changes in personality. Not associated with normal aging, dementia presents itself as a pathologic process such as Alzheimer's disease and Parkinson's disease. Although there are many different neurodegenerative disorders, only Alzheimer's disease and Parkinson's disease will be discussed.

Alzheimer's Disease

Alzheimer's disease (AD) is the most common cause of dementia in the elderly. The prevalence of AD will vary from those 60- to 64-years old to 1 to 40 percent over the age of 85 years. Women are slightly more affected than males with a ratio of 1.2 to 1.5. It is expected that as the Baby Boomers age, the number of patients diagnosed with AD will continue to increase.

When assessing AD, CT and MRI can be used to show diffuse cortical atrophy of the brain (Figure 2–13). Patients with AD demonstrate a marked degree of atrophy of the temporal lobe and hippocampus and parahippocampal gyrus.

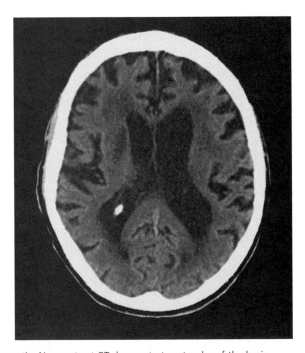

Figure 2–13 Dementia. Noncontrast CT demonstrates atrophy of the brain.

Parkinson's Disease

Parkinson's disease (PD) is another common progressive neurodegenerative disorder affecting approximately 1 percent of the population over 50 years of age. Patients with PD present with a narrowing of the pars compacta of the substantia nigra. This is best seen on a T2-weighted pulse sequence in MRI.

ADDITIONAL READING

Edelman, R. R., Hesselink, J. R., & Zlatkin, M. B. (1996). *Clinical magnetic resonance imaging.* 2nd ed. Vol. 1–2. Philadelphia: Saunders.

Grey, M. L., & Ailinani, J. M. (2003). *CT & MRI pathology: A pocket atlas.* New York: McGraw-Hill Professional.

Latchaw, R. E., Kucharczyk, J., & Moseley, M. E. (2005). *Imaging of the nervous system: Diagnostic and therapeutic applications.* Vol. 1–2. Philadelphia: Elsevier Mosby.

Stark, D.D., & Bradley, W. G. (1999). *Magnetic resonance imaging.* 3rd ed. Vol. 1–3. St. Louis: Mosby.

REFERENCES

Brain Injury Association of America (1986, February 22). *What is brain injury?* Retrieved January 9, 2006, from http://www.biausa.org/Pages/what_is_brain_injury.html

National Center for Injury Prevention and Control (2001). *Injury fact book 2001–2002.* Atlanta: Centers for Disease Control and Prevention.

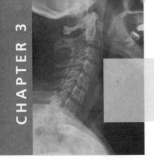

CHAPTER 3

Imaging of the Cervical Spine and Temporomandibular Joint

Diagnostic imaging assessment of the cervical spine is a challenge for even the experienced radiologist or practitioner. Patients may present with a broad spectrum of pathologies, including potentially catastrophic injuries requiring considerable interpretive prowess. While typical imaging modality use may identify most of the pathologies with which patients will present, particular attention to detail and use of multiple procedures may be required to identify complex or occult injuries. The ideal imaging tool would have perfect sensitivity and specificity to simplify this process, but no singularly superior diagnostic imaging tool exists. Rather, reasoning based on the patient history and most likely clinical scenarios dictate the decision making as to the diagnostic test of first choice and perhaps subsequently.

From a lateral view or in sagittal slices, gentle lordotic curves of the anterior and posterior margins of the vertebral bodies are to be present, forming a reference for continuity of the vertebrae and the connecting tissues. The anterior and posterior spinal lines allow basic comparison for vertebral positioning. The junctions of the laminae and spinous processes, representing the posterior border of the central canal, define the spinolaminar line and a third curvilinear reference. The vertebral bodies are rectangular with smooth, curved margins. The disk spaces are consistent and reveal like patterns of signal intensity on magnetic resonance imaging (MRI). The anterior aspects of spinous processes are in alignment, and the posterior tips of the spinous processes should be pointed in the same general direction (Mintz, 2004; Imhof and Fuchsjäger, 2002; Richards, 2005). The tips of the spinous processes form a fourth curvilinear reference, albeit used less frequently. The facet joints are paired at each level with the joint margins congruent and their spaces evident. The distance between the dens and anterior arch of the atlas remains consistent whether the image is in neutral or in a position of flexion or extension. Similarly, the aforementioned relationships of vertebra and disks remain relatively uniform throughout the spine with no disruption of the gradual curve regardless of position in the sagittal plane (Maus, 2002; Imhof and Fuchsjäger, 2002; Richards, 2005; Greenspan, 2000) (Figures 3–1 and 3–2).

From anteroposterior (AP) or in coronal plane views, the vertebral bodies are aligned in a relatively vertical column. The uncinate processes and, thus, the uncovertebral joints are clearly visible. The spinous processes are positioned in the midline. Features such as the facet joints, transverse processes, and the pedicles are often difficult to distinguish on plain radiographs, but are similarly aligned, if visible (Maus, 2002; Imhof and Fuchsjäger, 2002; Richards, 2005) (Figure 3–3).

Inspection of the upper cervical segments warrants particular attention to detail. The atlas is positioned with relative symmetry on the axis with no disruption in its

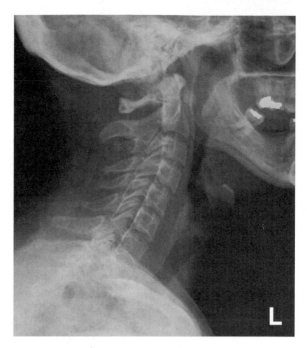

Figure 3–1 A lateral view conventional radiograph of the cervical spine in a 37-year-old woman.

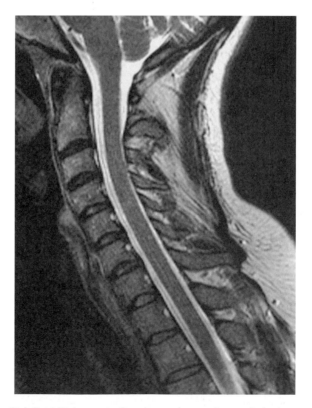

Figure 3–2 A sagittal slice MR demonstrating a normal-appearing cervical spine.

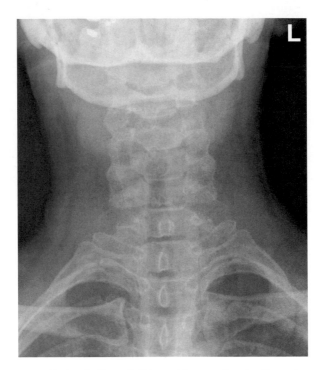

Figure 3–3 The same subject as in Figure 3–2 in an AP conventional radiograph.

osseous ring. The odontoid process is positioned symmetrically between the lateral masses of the atlas. The lateral C1-2 zygapophysial joint spaces are of equal height. The C2 spinous process is positioned in midline. In radiographs, the anterior and posterior arches of the atlas will be superimposed on the dens and are not to be interpreted as fracture lines (Maus, 2002; Imhof and Fuchsjäger, 2002; Richards, 2005). From a lateral view or in sagittal slices, the upper cervical soft tissue of the prevertebral region is to be inspected for normal lucency and signal intensities (Richards, 2005; Greenspan, 2000).

On T1-weighted MR images, the cerebrospinal fluid is of low signal intensity providing a contrast to the spinal cord, which is of intermediate signal. Osseous structures including the vertebral body, pedicles, laminae, and transverse and spinous processes demonstrate relatively high signal intensity. The two portions of the intervertebral disk can be discriminated to some degree as the nucleus pulposus is of intermediate signal and the surrounding annulus fibrosis of lower intensity (Figure 3–4). On T2-weighted images, the cord is low-intermediate signal and the cerebrospinal fluid is of high signal intensity, providing for a reference for the border of the cord. The vertebral body is at an intermediate level of intensity on T2-weighted images. The disks demonstrate contrast with high signal intensity from the nucleus pulposus and low signal from the annulus fibrosis. The nerve root sleeves are low-intermediate level of signal intensity, which again provides a reference for the interface of those tissues (Greenspan, 2000).

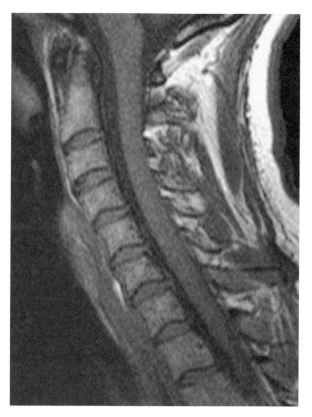

Figure 3–4 This T1-weighted MRI sagittal slice is a normal-appearing cervical spine. Note the similar alignment of features as described for conventional radiography along with the direct visualization of the soft tissues, including the intervertebral disks, spinal cord, and musculature.

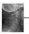 **RADIOGRAPHY**

Radiography of the cervical spine with AP and lateral views is a common method of assessing the integrity of the skeletal elements. Oblique posterior to anterior views are also occasionally chosen. While more sophisticated means are available and will be discussed later in this chapter, the continued use of radiography is in part due to factors of convenience for the patient and practitioner, rapidity of results, and relatively low cost. Simple radiographs perhaps offer the greatest benefit of quick screening for serious pathology given a history threatening disruption of typical skeletal relationships.

Pathologic conditions, such as disk herniations, tumors, or other soft tissue disorders potentially involving the neural elements, and some fractures have proven to be better demonstrated by other imaging modalities. As such, the sensitivity of radiography in detecting many pathologic conditions is relatively low. The prudent practitioner will recognize the limitations of such testing in not ruling out suspected pathologic conditions in the presence of negative results if other aspects of the clinical presentation remain consistent with syndromes for which radiography has low sensitivity.

Upper Cervical Spine

Owing to the critical nature of the integrity of the osteoligamentous structures of the craniovertebral junction, at least one additional view beyond the AP, lateral, and oblique views has traditionally been used to assess these elements. The odontoid (open-mouth) view has long been viewed as being particularly indicated in emergent care of patients with a history of trauma when fractures of this region are a possibility. Although such conventional radiography is still routinely used, a trend toward use of computed tomography (CT) as the introductory imaging modality in cervical spine trauma is evolving, particularly in patients at high risk for fracture. (Imhof and Fuchsjäger, 2002; Holmes and Akkinepalli, 2005; Van Goethem et al., 2005) (Figure 3–5).

Occipitocervical subluxation is occasionally survivable, particularly in children because of their ligamentous laxity. This injury is usually demonstrated on lateral view radiographs by the basion-dens interval (BDI) being greater than 12 millimeters (mm) (West, 2002). The BDI is measured between the anterior margin of the foramen magnum to the tip of the odontoid process.

Fractures of the posterior arch of the atlas are typically bilateral and are usually visible on lateral views. A burst fracture of the atlas (Jefferson fracture), which is usually the result of an axial load, may present with two to four fractures in the C1 ring. With an open-mouth view, lateral subluxation of the lateral masses may occur to indicate this

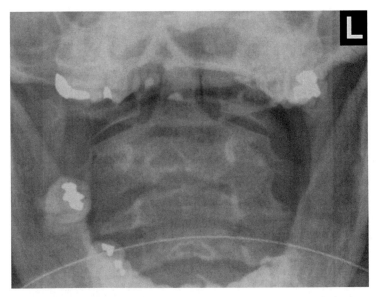

Figure 3–5 The subject is now imaged with the view focused on the upper cervical spine, particularly the odontoid process assessing for fracture.

injury. On a lateral view, often a clue of the shadow of prevertebral swelling will be present in the area and suggest the need for greater study (West, 2002; Harris, 2001).

Odontoid fractures are relatively common, accounting for 7 to 17 percent of all spinal fractures and are the most frequently missed on radiographic examination (West et al., 2003; Greenspan, 2000). In the absence of displacement of the fracture fragments, odontoid fractures may be overlooked on initial examination, requiring cautious interpretation by radiologists. Subtle findings such as tilting of the odontoid or cortical changes may be relatively inconspicuous. Again, the presence of the shadow of prevertebral swelling will raise the index of suspicion of such pathology (West et al., 2003; Greenspan, 2000) (Figure 3–6).

The system of classification of odontoid fractures by Anderson and D'Alonzo (1974) is most frequently used and is determined according to the location of the fracture line. Type I fractures involve only the tip of the odontoid process and are rare. Type II fractures are the most common as the fracture line is located at the base of the dens. If the fracture line extends through the upper body of C2, then classification as a type III is used. The orientation of the fracture lines of the type III odontoid fracture may be more visible on lateral view (West et al., 2003; Imhof and Fuchsjäger, 2002).

Occasionally, fractures of the C2 body may not reveal clear fracture lines, but an increase in the AP dimension of C2 suggested with a lateral radiograph implies fractures of the body and is known as the C2 fat sign (Pellei D, 2000; Jarolimek et al., 2004).

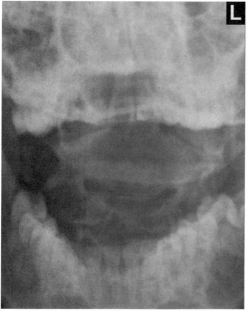
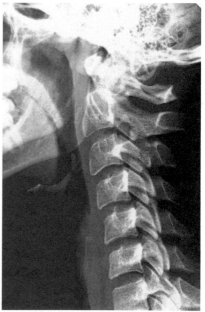

A   B

Figure 3–6 A. In this open-mouth view radiograph, discerning the fracture lines across the base of the odontoid process is not easily done. In this particular image, the inferior edge of the upper incisors could easily obstruct accurate examination of the odontoid. **B.** Similarly, in the lateral view radiograph, the multiple layers of osseous tissue present a challenge in viewing any potential injury of the odontoid process.

In addition to fractures of the upper cervical spine, acute injuries or degradation of the passive ligamentous restraints and other articular tissues are also of concern to the clinician and radiologist. While a history of trauma certainly raises suspicion of possible ligamentous injury, the destructive process associated with arthritides may also give rise to instability. Cervical subluxations are very common in individuals with rheumatoid arthritis (Kolen and Schmidt, 2002; Boden, 1993; Wolfe et al., 1987) with approximately 50 percent being asymptomatic (Cassar-Pullicino, 1999; Collins et al., 1991). Rehabilitation professionals are prudent to include physical examination procedures to detect findings suggestive of spinal cord compression in patients with rheumatoid arthritis. Among those signs associated with cord compression in rheumatoid arthritis are hyperreflexia, Babinksi's sign, objective muscle weakness, and gait disturbance (Reijnierse et al., 2001). Radiographic images are limited in their ability to detect instability of the craniovertebral region because of very incomplete image definition of soft tissues, but the disruption of normal skeletal relationships may indicate a loss of integrity of the interposed tissues. If radiography is chosen for the assessment of stability in rheumatoid arthritis, flexion views are recommended to enhance sensitivity (Kauppi and Neva, 1998). Multiple parameters to measure structural relationships may be used by radiologists. The accuracy of these measurements with radiography is, however, questionable due to, in part, the tissue changes associated with rheumatoid arthritis (Roche et al., 2002)

In patients with rheumatoid arthritis, atlantoaxial subluxation is the most common with subaxial subluxation being somewhat less frequent (Figure 3–7). The least frequent,

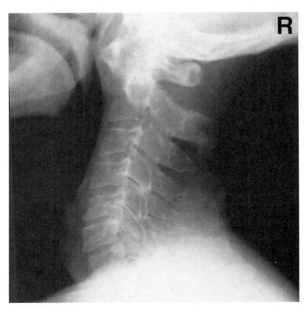

Figure 3–7 Subluxation of the atlantoaxial joint is a frequent finding with potentially serious consequences in those patients with rheumatoid arthritis. In this lateral view conventional radiograph, the radiologist estimated a 6-mm distance between the anterior arch of the atlas and the odontoid.

but most threatening, is basilar invagination, which is also termed cranial settling (Roche et al., 2002). Vertical instability due to erosion and degeneration may result in herniation of the cervical spine into the foramen magnum. Several investigators (Clark et al., 1989; Ranawat et al., 1979; Kauppi et al., 1990; Redlund-Johnell and Pettersson, 1984; McRae and Barnum, 1953; Chamberlain, 1939; McGregor, 1948; Wackenhelm, 1974) have devised indices to quantify basilar invagination and the attending risk of neurologic compromise, the details of which exceed the scope of this text. No single method with radiography has been determined to have the sensitivity and predictive value necessary to be considered clinically accurate (Riew et al., 2001). Thus, CT or MRI is recommended in any patient with rheumatoid arthritis and equivocal radiographs (Riew et al., 2001).

In addition to rheumatoid arthritis, other anomalies are associated with upper cervical instability. Down's syndrome, Marfan's disorder, and Ehler-Danlos syndrome have also been associated with such instability as a component of generalized ligamentous laxity (Pathria, 2005). Grisel's syndrome, in which upper cervical instability is frequently subsequent to an upper respiratory infection or retropharyngeal infection, has been observed mostly in children (Pathria, 2005; Okada et al., 2002; Haidar et al., 2005).

To measure atlantoaxial subluxation, the anterior atlanto-dens interval (AADI) has traditionally been used. In this measure, the spatial relationship between the odontoid process and anterior arch of the atlas has been used as a principal indicator of upper cervical stability. Before skeletal maturity, this value may be up to 4 to 5 mm. In adults and older children, a value of 3 mm is generally considered to be the upper limit of normal (Imhof and Fuchsjäger, 2002; Swischuk, 1999). Roche et al. (2002) proposes that 3 to 6 mm suggests transverse ligament damage and greater than 6 mm implies alar ligament injury.

Serial measures of AADI must be interpreted with caution. Over time, AADI may appear to improve, but collapse of the upper cervical segments may give the illusion of the AADI lessening because of the approximation of the occiput to C2 (Roche, 2002; Riew et al., 2001).

The posterior atlanto-dens interval (PADI) may be a more valuable measurement with a more accurate reflection of canal size and threat for neurologic compromise (Boden et al., 1993; Boden, 1994; Gurley and Bell, 1997; Cassar-Pullicino, 1999). The PADI is the distance between the posterior surface of the odontoid and the anterior margin of the posterior ring of the atlas. A PADI of 14 mm is considered the lower limit to avoid encroachment onto the spinal cord (Gurley and Bell, 1997; Zeidman and Tucker, 1994; Roche et al., 2002).

Radiographs in the neutral position will detect approximately one-half of atlantoaxial subluxations (Kauppi and Neva, 1998). Flexion positioning is considered more sensitive, but additional imaging beyond radiography is indicated for those patients particularly at risk for upper cervical instability (Roche et al., 2002).

Fractures of the pars interarticulares of C2 bilaterally or traumatic spondylolisthesis is also often demonstrable on a lateral view standard film. Some investigators equate this to the so-called hangman's fracture, but other investigators discriminate between the two injuries, noting differences from the mechanism of injury (Jaromilek et al., 2003; Effendi et al., 1981). Although the fractures may occur in the same region, the mechanism of injury with judicial hanging has typically been attributed to the mechanism of combined hyperextension and distraction, while spondylolisthesis is due to axial loading in either flexion or extension while being similarly traumatic (Jaromilek et al., 2003).

Other fractures of C2 may be categorized by the classification systems of Effendi et al. (1981) and Fujimura et al. (1996). Effendi type I fractures are of the ring of C2 with little to no displacement of the body. Type II fractures include displacement of the body and involvement of the C2–3 disk. Type III injuries are characterized by displacement of the body in an anterior position, but also by unilateral or bilateral subluxation or dislocation of the C2–3 zygapophysial joints (Jaromilek et al., 2003; Effendi et al., 1981).

The Fujimura classification system consists of four types. Type I is the teardrop fracture; named for the wedge-shaped avulsion fracture fragment from traction of the anterior longitudinal ligament from sudden, violent hyperextension (Jaromilek et al., 2003; Fujimura et al., 1996). Type II fracture is transversely oriented through the body but caudal to the previously mentioned type III odontoid fracture. Type III fracture is a burst fracture with comminution of the body. A sagittal or parasagittal fracture from a point lateral to the dens to the inferior surface of C2 is considered a type IV injury (Fujimura et al., 1996).

Lower Cervical Spine

Avulsion fracture of a lower cervical or first thoracic spinous process (clay shoveler's fracture) is readily demonstrated by a lateral view radiograph. This particular injury has been reported to be from forceful contraction of the cervical spine musculature into flexion against tense posterior elements. This fracture is usually without compromise of ligamentous stability (Imhof and Fuchsjäger, 2002; Matar et al., 2000; Dellestable and Gaucher, 1998).

The teardrop fracture, as described above for C2, also occurs in similar fashion in the lower cervical spine but due to flexion-compression force causing a fracture line and separating a teardrop-shaped fragment of bone off the anterior-inferior aspect of the vertebral body. Significant ligamentous injury is often associated with teardrop fractures with concurrent neurologic compromise (Imhof and Fuchsjäger, 2002; Richards, 2005).

By similar mechanism, wedge compression fractures of the lower cervical spine can occur and may be accompanied by subluxation anteriorly (Richards, 2005; Imhof and Fuchsjäger, 2002).

Fractures of the articular pillar have been reported to occur due to axial load with combined flexion and rotation and are perhaps best viewed in lateral or oblique view radiographs, although CT offers a superior visualization (Shanmuganathan et al., 1996; Imhof and Fuchsjäger, 2002).

Similarly, spondylolysis of the cervical spine, although less known than in the lumbar region, may also be revealed on radiographs (Redla et al., 1999). Occasionally, the displacement in the form of spondylolisthesis (anterior) or retrolisthesis (posterior) may occur. In both cases, the translatory displacement of the vertebra is the key feature, with the threat of encroachment onto the spinal cord being a concern that may require additional imaging (Maus, 2002; Kopacz and Connolly, 1999) (Figure 3–8).

Instability may also be suggested with displacement of typical vertebra from the previously described alignment due to traumatic or degenerative processes. This may

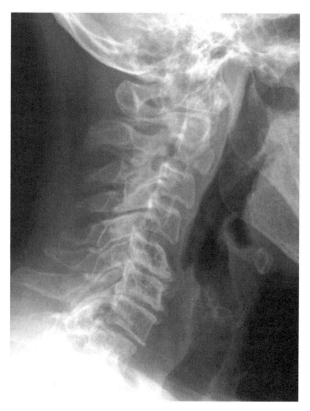

Figure 3–8 In this lateral view radiograph from a 74-year-old man, surrounding the degenerative change most evident at C5–6 is anterolisthesis of C4–5 and C6–7.

be demonstrated to a greater degree if flexion/extension radiographs are utilized to reveal relative greater movement at a segment and the suspect integrity of the passive restraint mechanisms (Lewis et al., 1991; Pollack et al., 2001). This phenomenon may be demonstrated by lateral radiographs as translation of the anterior margin of one vertebral body more than 3 to 5 mm beyond the subjacent vertebral body or more than 11 degrees angulation between adjacent end plates (Roche et al., 2001; Richards, 2005; Imhof and Fuchsjäger, 2002). Spinal canal diameter, however, may be a better predictor of neurologic problems with a normal sagittal diameter of 14 to 23 mm from C3–7. Such examination is undertaken only with long-term follow-up of whiplash-type injuries and is specifically avoided in the acutely injured spine (Imhof and Fuchsjäger, 2002; Pathria, 2005; Richards, 2005). If multiple levels of instability are involved, as may occur with rheumatoid arthritis, a stepladder deformity may be noted on lateral radiographs (Roche et al., 2001) (Figures 3–9 and 3–10).

Subluxation of a zygapophysial joint or a "jumped" or "perched" facet is often readily visible on a standard lateral view as indicated by the disruption in typical alignment of the spinous processes, the articular processes, and the vertebral bodies. This injury is

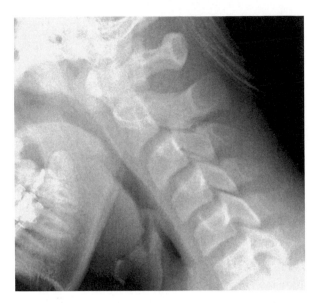

Figure 3–9 In this flexed position of the cervical spine, there is approximately 3 mm anterior displacement of the C2 vertebra on C3.

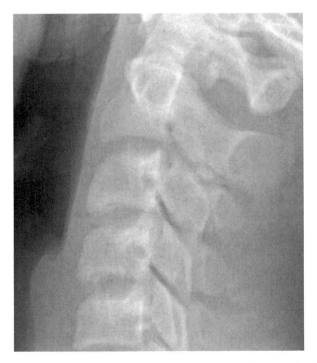

Figure 3–10 Subsequent positioning in extension reduces the forward displacement of C2 on C3.

often due to a flexion-distraction mechanism and is usually associated with neurologic deficit (Imhof and Fuchsjäger, 2002; Lingawi, 2001; Andreshak and Dekutoski, 1997; Manaster and May, 2002).

Perhaps most routinely for patients of middle age and beyond presenting with position or movement-dependent axial or periscapular pain, suspicion must be greatest for mechanical pain syndromes associated with degenerative changes. Lateral view radiographs may suggest loss of disk height, subchondral sclerosis of the zygapophysial joints, and osteophyte formation about the vertebral body-disk, uncovertebral joint, and zygapophysial joint margins. The correlation of such findings to painful syndromes is not definitive as similar observations have been made in asymptomatic populations (Roh et al., 2005; Maus, 2002; Gore, 2001).

Projection of the oblique-anterior view may allow the observer greater ability to view the intervertebral foramina of the cervical spine. Radiography with this view may be most appropriate with suspicion of bony compromise of the foramina (Maus, 2002).

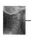 COMPUTED TOMOGRAPHY

CT is most often utilized for cervical spine examination in the assessment of potential fractures due to a primary ability to display bony integrity. Given its limitations in demonstrating soft tissue features, CT may not be the modality of choice when soft tissue imaging is of primary interest. With the addition of injected contrast, CT myelography (CTM) is considered an excellent method of imaging because of its sensitivity in revealing information concerning the spinal cord and nerve roots.

Guidelines relative to risk factors have evolved as to the recommended imaging modality in emergent care situations (Goldberg et al., 2001; Hanson et al., 2000; Steill et al., 2001; Vandemark, 1990). The greater sensitivity of CT in detecting cervical spine fractures frequently warrants utilization of CT over conventional radiography. Patients viewed as low risk for fracture are examined with radiography, but those noted to be at high risk are routed directly to CT (Nguyen and Clark, 2005; Grogan et al., 2005; Holmes et al., 2005; Van Goethem et al., 2005). The presence of multiple risk factors for life-threatening injury in traumatized persons, such as high-energy trauma, other fractures or altered consciousness, specifically indicate the need for more sophisticated imaging.

Similarly, considerably higher rates of upper cervical fractures have been noted in elderly patients, increasing the indication for CT scanning for older patients presenting with trauma (Hanson et al., 2000; Lomoschitz et al., 2004; Muller et al., 1999). Interestingly, the use of CT in these patients is ultimately proving cost effective as compared to radiography (Grogan et al., 2005; Van Goethem et al., 2005; Berlin, 2003).

Multiple studies (Nguyen and Clark, 2005; Grogan et al., 2005; Holmes et al., 2005; Van Goethem et al., 2005; Holmes and Akkinepalli, 2005) have indicated CT to be superior to radiography in detecting fractures of the cervical spine, even small fractures (Mintz, 2004) (Figures 3–11 to 3–16). Except by secondary signs (i.e., facet joint widening, anterior vertebral body translation), CT does not show ligamentous or other soft tissue injury (Kaiser et al., 1998). In the case of trauma, patients are often evaluated with radiographs

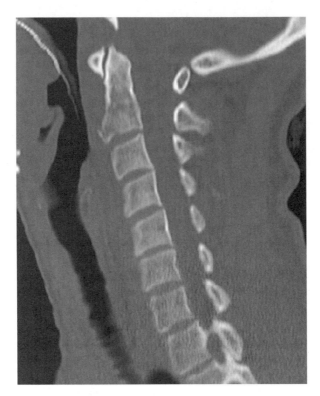

Figure 3–11 In this sagittal reconstruction CT, a teardrop fracture of the C2 vertebral body is demonstrated.

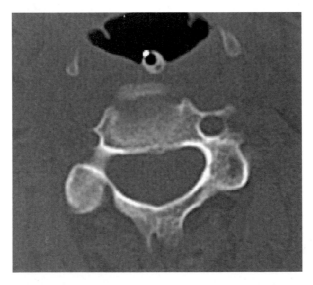

Figure 3–12 In the axial image, the size and displacement of the fracture fragment from the lower anterior vertebral body is further appreciated.

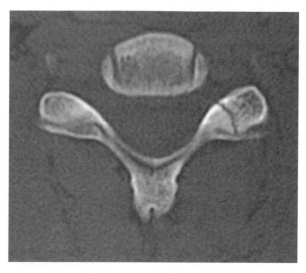

Figure 3–13 The axial CT image of the C6 vertebra in this image reveals a fracture of the zygapophysial joint surface.

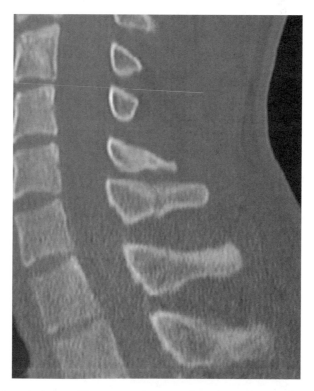

Figure 3–14 This sagittal plane CT reconstruction upon close observation reveals a nondisplaced C7 spinous process fracture.

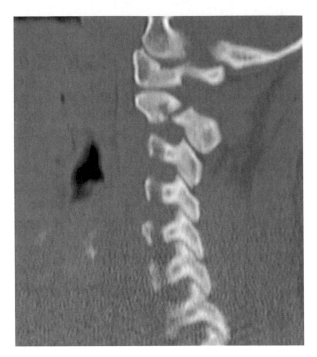

Figure 3–15 This sagittal CT reconstruction reveals injury to C2 known as a hangman's fracture.

in conjunction with CT. This combination of diagnostic imaging tests is considered highly sensitive to detecting fractures, even more than CT alone (Widder et al., 2004).

In addition to the axial views, radiologists often consider obtaining sagittal and coronal reconstructions essential to provide information about cord compression and facet dislocation (Mink, 2003).

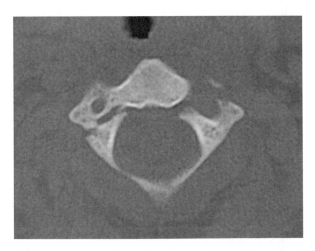

Figure 3–16 The axial image reveals the bilateral fracture pattern associated with a hangman's fracture.

Occipital condyle fractures are readily seen on CT, but are not well visualized with radiography because of the superimposition of neighboring bony features complicating visualization. These fractures are best identified with a high-resolution, thin-slice (1 to 2 mm) CT scans (Capuano et al., 2004; Leone et al., 2000). Occipital condyle fractures typically occur from impact directly onto the head. Often patients presenting acutely with the possibility of these injuries may not be able to participate in open-mouth standard films because of other factors such as loss of consciousness or intubation (Capuano et al., 2004; West, 2002; Leone et al., 2000; Tuli et al., 1997; Hanson et al., 2002) (Figure 3–17).

According to the classification system of Anderson and Montesano (1988), a type I occipital condyle fracture is a comminuted impaction fracture usually from a blow to the top of head, yielding a stable injury usually. A type II fracture is also typically from an impact to the top of the head, but the fracture fragment extends into the occipital bone. Although usually stable, instability can occur if the fracture fragment is displaced. A type III injury is a wedge-shaped avulsion fracture involving the alar ligament on the medial aspect of the occipital condyles. This is frequently associated with occipitocervical instability (West, 2002).

Tuli et al. (1997) proposes a slightly different classification system of occipital condyle fractures. Type I is nondisplaced. Type IIa is characterized by displacement of the fracture fragment, but no ligamentous injury. Type IIb is a displaced fracture with ligamentous injury and is unstable.

C1 fractures are best visualized with CT, particularly if the fracture line is through the lateral mass, which may be obscured on radiographs. Fracture lines of the posterior arch are easily visualized with CT, and the number of fracture fragments of burst (Jefferson) fractures can readily be determined. CT is especially appropriate for trauma patients with a high index of suspicion and specially formatted, high-quality images may be required (West et al., 2002; Harris, 2001) (Figure 3–18).

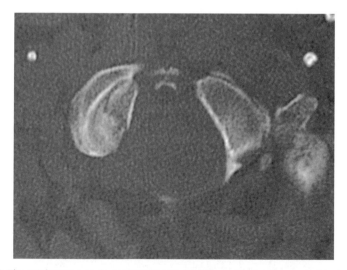

Figure 3–17 The axial CT image demonstrates an occipital condyle fracture; such injuries are difficult to identify with radiography.

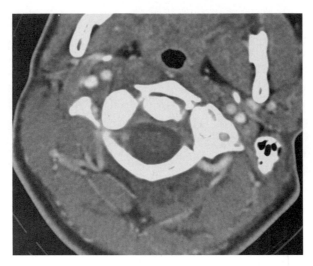

Figure 3–18 An axial CT bone windows view of a Jefferson fracture in a 15-year- old boy. Note the quadripartite configuration of the atlas with fractures anterior and posterior to the lateral masses bilaterally.

Thin-slice CT is preferable for patients at high risk for fractures of the dens. Type II fractures at the base of the dens (as discussed in the preceding section) may be elusive on radiographs if no displacement occurs, but are better detected with CT (West et al., 2002; Harris, 2001; Imhof and Fuchsjäger, 2002) (Figures 3–19 and 3–20). In addition to fractures, CT provides for a more detailed view than radiography in demonstrating erosion of the dens and facet joints, typical of rheumatoid disease (Kolen and Schmidt, 2002) (Figures 3–21 and 3–22).

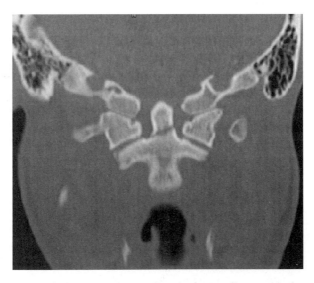

Figure 3–19 In this coronal plane CT reconstruction, the fracture line near the base of the odontoid is clearly evident.

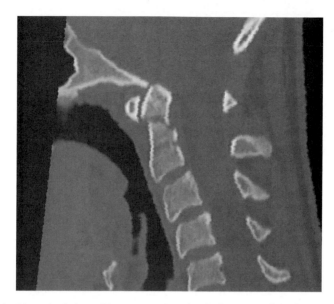

Figure 3–20 In this sagittal plane CT reconstruction, the displacement of the fracture with reference to possible encroachment on the spinal cord is evident.

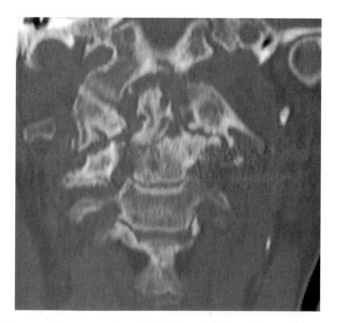

Figure 3–21 The coronal reconstruction of this CT reveals advanced erosive changes of the upper cervical spine, particularly of the odontoid process and the atlantoaxial joints.

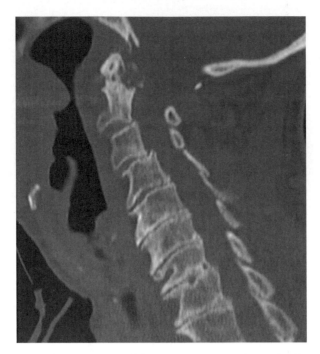

Figure 3–22 In the sagittal reconstruction of the same image series, the erosive changes are again evident along with tendency toward subluxation of C3-4. Degenerative change is evident throughout the cervical spine.

Recently, multidetector row CT has evolved to allow sophisticated three-dimensional imaging in any plane and has been reported to be particularly effective in detecting fractures of the traumatized cervical spine (Li and Fishman, 2003). The capability of thin-slice, high-definition multiplane reconstructions also proves particularly valuable in examining the obliquely oriented intervertebral foramina for possible lateral stenosis. Even prior to the multidetector row units came into use, spiral CT allowed for best examination for bony stenosis from the zygapophysial and uncovertebral joints (Mintz, 2004; Kaiser et al., 1998) (Figure 3–23).

CTM and MRI are both used in the examination for suspected stenosis (Maus, 2002; Stafira et al., 2003), and CTM is superior to standard myelography (Kaiser et al., 1998) in evaluating possible osseous encroachment from spondylosis. The lack of soft tissue imaging by CT is negated in large part by the addition of contrast to allow assessment of the disk–thecal sac and thecal sac–ligamentum flavum interfaces (Maus, 2002). CTM is particularly of value in examining nerve root origins (Mink, 2003). The invasiveness and potential for complications of CTM may, however, relegate it to a second line of decision making for many physicians and be particularly indicated in patients with concerns of significant prior history of injury or surgery, those with congenital complexities, or those for whom imminent surgery is a consideration (Mink, 2003) (Figures 3–24 and 3–25).

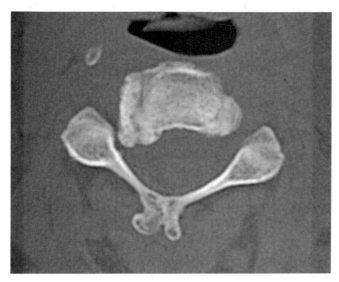

Figure 3–23 In this axial CT image, osteophytic growth has significantly narrowed the intervertebral foramen.

CT has limited application in examination of tumors, but may be required with neoplasms to determine the chondroid and osteoid matrix of the lesions (Mink, 2003).

The jumped or "perched" facet described under conventional radiography is also visible on CT by the telltale "naked" or "uncovered" facet sign (Imhof and Fuchsjäger, 2002; Lingawi, 2001; Andreshak and Dekutoski, 1997) (Figure 3–26 to 3–28).

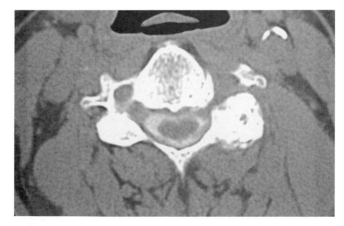

Figure 3–24 In this axial image of the post-myelogram CT scan, note the absence of contrast filling the nerve root.

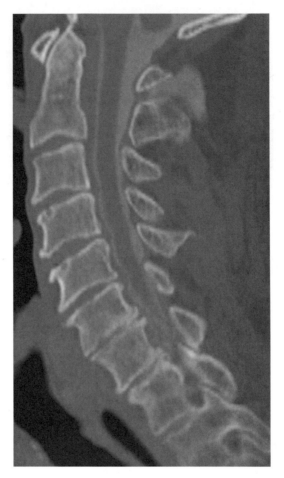

Figure 3–25 In the sagittal reconstructions of the post-myelogram CT scan, small indentations of the contrast material representing spondylitic bars extending posteriorly from the vertebral bodies are evident, although no definite disk herniations.

 ## MAGNETIC RESONANCE IMAGING

MRI allows clear visualization of the ligementous, neural, diskal, muscular, and other soft tissue features along with the osseous structures typically required in clinical decision making. Views are usually obtained with slices in sagittal and axial sequences.

MRI is usually not the primary method of fracture detection, but is the preferred imaging modality to address suspicion of associated ligamentous injury and the assessment of the status of nearby neural tissues (Jinkins, 2001; Wilmink, 1999). Injury to ligaments is likely to produce changes in spatial relationships and signal intensity. The

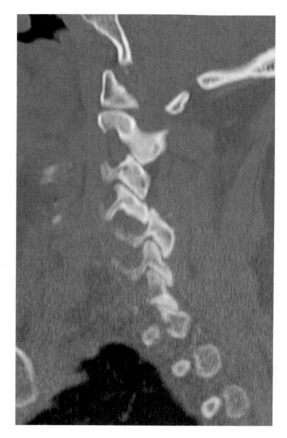

Figure 3–26 A sagittal CT reconstruction in a 61-year-old woman demonstrating a facet lock or jumped facet at C4–5.

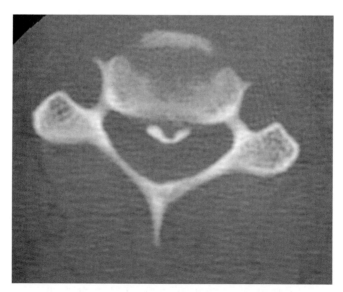

Figure 3–27 The axial image of the cervical spine reveals ossification of the posterior longitudinal ligament. *Image courtesy of Travis Fromwiller, MD, Department of Radiology, Medical College of Wisconsin, Milwaukee, Wisconsin.*

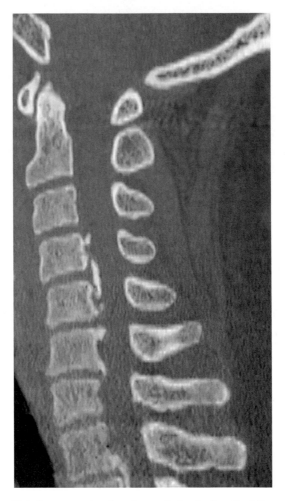

Figure 3–28 The sagittal plane reconstruction demonstrates the length of the ossification of the ligament. *Image courtesy of Travis Fromwiller, MD, Department of Radiology, Medical College of Wisconsin, Milwaukee, Wisconsin.*

longitudinal ligaments and ligamentum flavum appear as thin linear bands of low signal intensity on all sequences. Acute gross rupture will be represented by discontinuity and hemorrhage, which will often be accompanied by altered alignment (Figure 3–29). Less overt ligament injury will typically demonstrate irregularity, thickening, and greater signal intensity associated with inflammation (Pathria, 2005). T1-weighted images often are best to identify hemorrhage, while T2-weighted images or other special sequences will often reveal other inflammatory processes associated with ligamentous injury, including spinal cord injury (Imhof and Fuchsjäger, 2002; Pathria, 2005; Jinkins, 2001).

Further, spinal cord injury can be characterized, identifying and distinguishing between cord edema, hemorrhage, or transection, which is of major prognostic significance. Generally, patients demonstrating intramedullary hemorrhage have a worse prognosis than

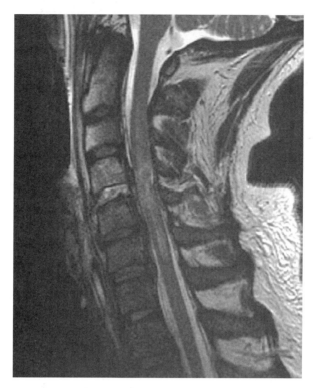

Figure 3–29 This sagittal section T2-weighted MRI reveals major disruption of the C4–5 segment in this 23-year-old man. Increased signal intensity is evident in the intradiskal space along with injury to the posterior longitudinal ligament. Edema within the spinal cord is evident spanning multiple levels around the injury.

those who do not, and patients with findings consistent with edema in the absence of hemorrhage often sustain considerable functional improvement (Figure 3–30) (Grabb and Pang, 1994; Hayashi et al., 1995; Stark and Bradley, 1999; Tewari et al., 2005). Further, the immediate identification of spinal cord pathology with MRI allows critical decisions which can affect long-term outcomes (Tewari et al., 2005; Papadopoulos et al., 2005). While spinal cord injury without radiographic abnormality (SCIWORA) may account for up to 12 percent of all cases of spinal cord injury, MRI typically identifies the soft tissue injury not represented on radiography or CT from which this phenomenon was originally described (Tewari et al., 2005).

For whiplash-associated disorders, MRI has not consistently demonstrated remarkable findings in the absence of neurologic involvement. Several studies have failed to discriminate significant findings in patients with whiplash-associated disorders from nontraumatized individuals (Steinberg et al., 2005; Borchgrevink et al., 1997; Karlsborg et al., 1997; Ronnen et al., 1996; Voyvodic et al., 1997). Thus, MRI is usually not performed unless there are signs or symptoms of cord injury or radiculopathy (Kaiser et al., 1998). Particular involvement of the upper cervical ligamentous structures as identified on MRI has been suggested

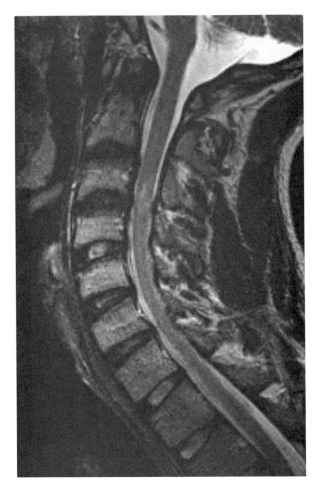

Figure 3–30 A sagittal section T2-weighted MRI of the cervical spine in a 21-year-old man. Note the signal change present within the spinal cord approximating the C3–4 levels, which is consistent with edema and a spinal cord contusion. This individual was particularly susceptible to injury because of congenital stenosis.

as a causative factor in persistent pain subsequent to whiplash (Kaale et al., 2005; Krakenes et al., 2002, 2003). This theory has not gained widespread support within the field of radiologic study of the spine on account of questionable interobserver agreement and other methodologic concerns (Kwan, 2003; Pape, 2004; Wilmink, 2001). Findings such as prevertebral edema, however, are noteworthy and typically stimulate a vigorous diagnostic process considering fracture or instability (Figure 3–31).

MRI best demonstrates many of the effects of rheumatoid arthritis on the cervical spine, including erosions of the upper cervical segments, the presence or absence of compression of the brainstem or spinal cord, encroachment on the subarachnoid space, pannus formation, and the altered spatial relationships (Reijnierse et al., 2001; Kolen and Schmidt, 2002) (Figure 3–32).

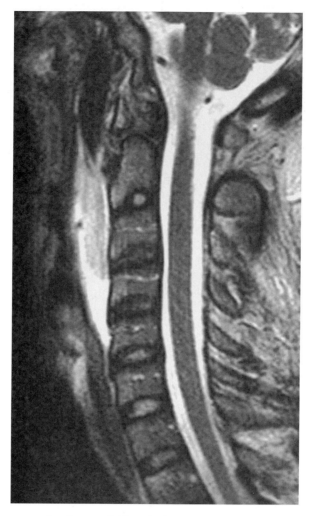

Figure 3–31 The outstanding feature of this sagittal section T2-weighted MR image is the increased signal intensity consistent with edema from soft tissue injury. The presence of such findings warrants particular caution to examine scrupulously for the presence of fractures.

Degenerative changes of the cervical spine, specifically involving the intervertebral disks, may be identified by loss of disk height, loss of disk signal from desiccation, annular fissures, diskal calcification, osteophytosis, reactive end plate changes, and displacement. The effects of this cascade may result in narrowing of the associated intervertebral foramina. MRI is the most sensitive option in detecting disk degeneration. T2-weighted images are more sensitive than T1-weighted images in detecting loss of water or proteoglycan content of the disks (Abdulkarim et al., 2003).

The presence of apparent pathology must always be correlated to the clinical presentation due to the frequency of findings in asymptomatic individuals. Changes consistent

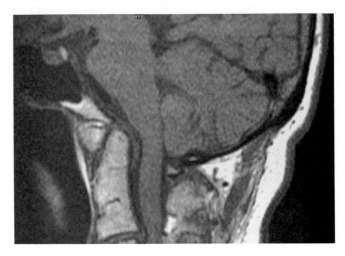

Figure 3–32 A T1-weighted MRI revealing basilar invagination. Observe the protrusion of the odontoid process into the foramen magnum and the resulting displacement of the brainstem.

with degeneration are routinely found in asymptomatic persons beyond their fifth decades (Figure 3–33). Several investigators (Boden et al., 1990; Teresi et al., 1987; Matsumoto et al., 1998; Ernst et al., 2005; Siivola et al., 2002) have found evidence of disk herniation and degeneration, annular tears, and foraminal stenosis in asymptomatic middle-aged populations. Clear extrusions and compression of neural elements are more directly associated with the presence of symptoms (Ernst et al., 2005; Siivola et al., 2002) (Figures 3–34 and 3–35). Radiologists may have difficulty in determining the age of a pathoanatomic lesion such as a disk herniation as they are often accompanied by degenerative changes such as disk desiccation, loss of disk height, and osseous ridging (Kaiser, 1998), which limits the ability to interpret the causality of the lesion with a painful syndrome. Low signal T2-weighted images are well correlated with histologic degeneration of the disk, including loss if turgor, subsequent loss of height, bulging of the annulus, and ultimately both vertical and AP narrowing of the foramina (Mink, 2003).

MRI best defines the degree of central spinal stenosis, whether caused by central disk herniation or broad-based osseous ridging (Figure 3–36). Osteophytes arising from the posterolateral uncovertebral joints and overgrowth of the posterior facet joints contribute to central and foraminal stenosis (Kaiser et al., 1998; Mehdorn et al., 2005). T2-weighted images are best for evaluating for possible central canal and thecal sac compromise by osteophyte or disk encroachment as the cord appears medium intensity with the cerebrospinal fluid appearing bright (Kaiser, 1998; Mehdorn et al., 2005). With the use of MRI, myelopathy secondary to intrinsic cord disease can easily be distinguished from myelopathy secondary to compressive disease. A positive correlation has been demonstrated between the cross-sectional area of the spinal cord as measured by MRI and the severity of myelopathy along with recovery after decompression (Okada et al., 1993; Fujiwara et al., 1998; Suda et al., 2003). Methodologies have been proposed for

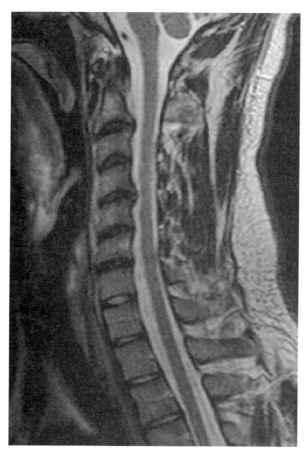

Figure 3–33 In this sagittal slice of a T2-weighted MRI of the cervical spine in a 44-year-old man, changes typical of the age are evident including the decreased signal intensity of the cervical intervertebral disks, bulging disks (without herniation), and osteophytic lipping at the disk and vertebral body margins.

qualitatively assessing spinal canal diameter, but their reliability has not been established (Stafira et al., 2003). *Myelomalacia* refers to the findings associated with degenerative change progressively threatening the spinal cord. Early MRI findings include a poorly defined area of increased signal intensity within the cord on T2-weighted images possibly due to associated edema, vascular stasis, and gliosis; T1-weighted images are typically normal. Prolonged compression can result in cystic necrosis and cavitation of the gray matter. Syrinxes may form and the cord may atrophy (Mink et al., 2003). In addition to the nonspecific complaints of widespread aches, rehabilitation professionals must be alert to the physical findings resulting from compressive disease including sensory changes, unsteady gait, hyperreflexia, Romberg's sign, Hoffman's sign, myoclonus, Babinski's sign, spasticity, disruption of bowel and bladder functions, and weakness in at least one limb (Heffez et al., 2004; Mehdorn et al., 2005).

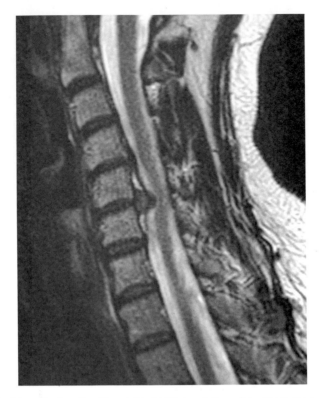

Figure 3–34 In this sagittal section T2-weighted MRI, herniation of the C5–6 disk is evident.

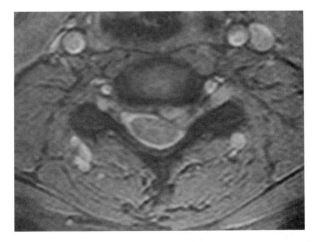

Figure 3–35 In this axial T2-weighted MR image, the effect of displacing the spinal cord and cervical nerve root is visible.

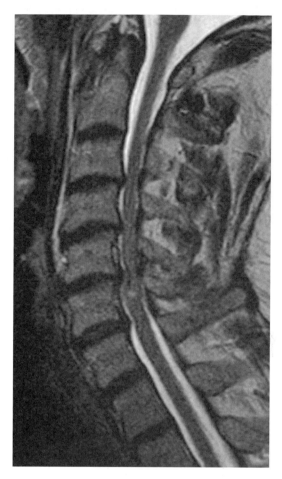

Figure 3–36 A sagittal view T2-weighted MRI revealing advanced degenerative change resulting in central spinal canal stenosis. Note the absence of signal from the cerebrospinal fluid in the areas of osteophytic growth and disk bulging.

MRI is the most sensitive and specific imaging modality for the diagnosis of spinal infection (Kaiser et al., 1998; Rothman et al., 1996; Tali, 2004). Radiography and CT demonstrable bone destruction may lag behind clinical infection by 2 to 10 weeks, which may prove critical to patient management (Maiuri et al., 1997; Perrone et al., 1994; Hopkinson et al., 2001). On T1-weighted images, the infectious process will cause decreased signal intensity and a loss of definition of the end plates, leading to less distinction between the vertebral body and the disk. There may be interruption of the continuity, typically present at the cortical margins. Further, enhancement upon administration of contrast is a hallmark of infection, allowing the extent of the infectious process and any compromise of the cord to be identified. On T2-weighted images, signal intensity is increased in the vertebral body and disk. With the abscess hyperintense on T2-weighted images, the infection may be difficult to differentiate from the adjacent cerebrospinal fluid and fat (both bright) (Mink et al., 2003; Tali, 2004; Stosic-Opincal et al., 2004). An important feature to discriminate an infectious process from neoplastic disease is the tendency for infectious processes to traverse disks (Khanna et al., 2002) (Figure 3–37).

MRI is the best method for consideration of primary and secondary cord tumors. Tumors of the spine are usually classified by location: extradural, intradural-extramedullary, and intramedullary. The location of the tumors and their signal characteristics allow for accurate diagnosis, the full scope of which exceeds this work. MRI is the investigative method of choice for suspected neoplasm. The level, location, and specific characteristics of the tumor can usually be visualized from MR images (Kaiser et al., 1998; Perrin and Laxton, 2004). Metastases to the bone generally present with low signal intensity on T1-weighted images and high signal intensity on T2-weighted images (Figure 3–38).

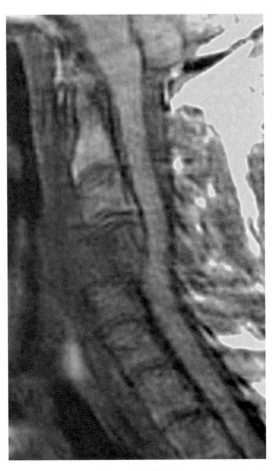

Figure 3–37 Although this image is somewhat degraded by motion artifact, involvement of the vertebral body of C4 with findings consistent with osteomyelitis is readily apparent. Images degraded from patient motion are frequently a challenge for the physician undertaking interpretation.

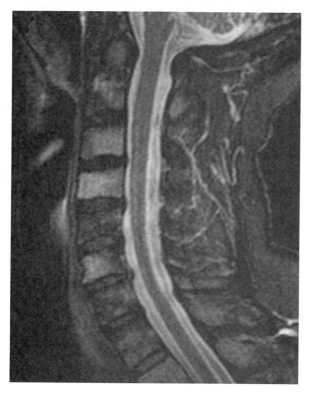

Figure 3–38 In this sagittal section T2-weighted MRI, diffuse metastatic disease is seen in multiple cervical vertebrae as highlighted by the increased signal intensity.

Additionally, the change of signal with osteoporosis typically does not affect the pedicles, which are frequently involved with neoplastic disease. The most common metastases are from the lung, prostate, breast, and kidneys and from melanoma (Karagianis et al., 2003; Perrin and Laxton, 2004). Administration of contrast is often undertaken when unenhanced images fail to reveal findings consistent with the clinical presentation (Loughrey et al., 2000). The cervical spine has a lower frequency of neoplastic lesions than the other regions of the spine (Perrin and Laxton, 2004; Loughrey et al., 2000).

MRI demonstrates the plaques associated with multiple sclerosis in the spinal cord, often in the cervical region. Standard T2-weighted images and gadolinium-enhanced T1-weighted images are the most frequently chosen methods. The plaques appear as bright images, expand the cord, and can be multiple during active stages of the disease (Mink et al., 2003; Arnold and Matthews, 2002). Similarly, MRI demonstrates the diffuse lesion characteristic of transverse myelitis with the cord expanded acutely (Mink et al., 2003). Gadolinium enhancement of the spinal cord consistent with inflammation and the absence of compressive disease are important findings toward the diagnosis of transverse myelitis (Transverse Myelitis Consortium Working Group, 2002). The imaged lesions associated with transverse myelitis generally involve more than two-thirds of the cord cross-sectional area on the axial images and may extend across multiple segments as viewed on the sagittal slices, involving considerably greater volume of the cord than that usually demonstrated by multiple sclerosis (Chin, 2002; Kalita et al., 2002) (Figure 3–39).

Primary motor neuron diseases directly affect the spinal cord. MRI, with T2-weighted images, can demonstrate the lateral tract degeneration accompanying diseases such as primary amyotrophic lateral sclerosis and primary lateral sclerosis (Mink, 2003). Magnetic resonance imaging may show high signal intensity in the corticospinal tracts (Chan et al., 1999).

MRI may be required in the advancing stages of ankylosing spondylitis due to the ability to image soft tissues, particularly cord involvement. Patients with ankylosing spondylitis are also particularly susceptible to fractures, which may require more than radiography to assess the possible presence of fractures and instability, particularly in those with neurologic signs or symptoms (Pedrosa et al., 2002; Nakstad et al., 2004).

Dynamic MRI (Mink, 2003) has been found to change the magnitude of epidural space, affect the volume of disk displacement, and affect foraminal space, but correlating these

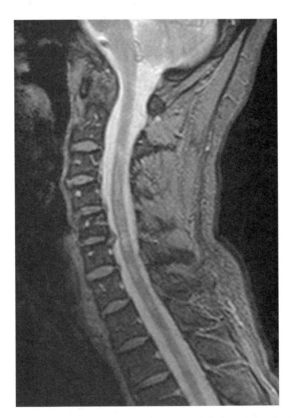

Figure 3–39 This T2-weighted MRI with contrast shows areas of altered signal within the spinal cord consistent with plaque lesions typical of multiple sclerosis. The plaques are not contrast enhanced, suggesting the image was not captured during a flare of the disease.

changes to pain origin remains elusive. Trials by Chen et al. (2003) and Muhle et al. (1998) have demonstrated greater sensitivity to detecting impingement upon neural structures.

Foraminal narrowing lesions have been missed on MRI and are usually of osteophytic disease in origin (Yousem et al., 1991). Particular caution may be warranted when evaluating cervical foramina by MRI and findings should be compared with those on oblique plain radiographic films. Thin-section gradient echo axial MR has been observed to cause an overestimation of the degree of foraminal narrowing, often related to patient motion (Kaiser et al., 1998).

 ## DISKOGRAPHY

Diskography maintains an important role in diagnosis of diskogenic cervical spine pain, but the results demand cautious interpretation. MRI is often capable of identifying a painful disk, but high false-positive and false-negative rates have been recognized using MRI in comparison to the reproduction of symptoms with discography (Parfenchuck and Janssen, 1994; Zheng et al., 2004). Thus, given the markedly different anatomy of the cervical disk in comparison to the lumbar disk, the dispersal of the contrast administered during cervical diskography is of little importance. Filling of uncovertebral clefts or recesses with contrast in CT diskography is generally considered typical of a maturing disk and must be differentiated from an annular tear. Thus, annular tears can be missed by MRI, while the source of cervical pain is often not reliably identified (Schellhas et al., 1996). For patients with equivocal MRI results or poor correlation of images to clinical signs and symptoms, cervical diskography offers the only test to combine anatomic and physiologic data, but its use remains relatively infrequent (Mink, 2003).

The key issue with diskography persists with judging the patient's response in attempting to identify concordant pain. Replication of the primary complaint of pain may be the objective, but may be complicated by segmental overlap of pain distribution (Mink, 2003). More recently, investigators have mapped pain patterns of disks in two studies (Slipman et al., 2005; Schellhas et al., 2000) with relatively good consistency. The reader is referred to those studies for elaboration of diskogenic pain patterns. Although generally considered safe, the invasive nature of the procedure is not without risk; complication rates of 0.6 to 2.48 percent have been reported (Grubb and Kelly, 2000; Zeidman et al., 1995; Guyer et al., 1997). The primary value of diskography in addition to identifying a surgical target has been proposed to be in determining on which level surgery is not to be performed (Bogduk, 2002).

 ## IMAGING OF THE TEMPOROMANDIBULAR JOINT

Knowledge of imaging results of the temporomandibular joint (TMJ) is imperative for rehabilitation professionals engaged in caring for patients with dysfunction. Owing to the complex anatomy of this region, the choice of imaging is highly dependent upon the suspected pathology.

Radiography is of relatively little value in diagnosis of temporomandibular disorders on account of the small size of the joint, the dense osseous surrounding tissues, and widely varying morphology of the condyle and fossa (Dias et al., 2005). Radiography is limited to assessment of the overall amplitude of joint movements without providing detail as to underlying pathology (Abolmaali et al., 2004).

CT is the preferred method for primary investigation of potential osseous deformities, particularly three-dimensional CT (Gorgu et al., 1999). CT is precise in allowing the cortical bone to be visualized and is particularly of value when investigating possible maxillofacial trauma, congenital skeletal anomalies, or neoplastic disease with destruction of the condyle (Abolmaali et al., 2004) (Figure 3–40). Simlarly, three-dimensional CT clearly demonstrates ankylosis when present (Gorgu et al., 2000). Accuracy of CT-estimated bony measures has been confirmed in comparison to cadaveric specimens (Honda et al., 2004).

Imaging of the TMJ will frequently involve MRI owing to its superior ability to image soft tissues including the articular disk, which is frequently involved with temporomandibular dysfunction (Abolmaali et al., 2004; Babadag et al., 2004). Location, movement, and morphology of the disk may all be assessed on MRI with the mandible in closed and open positions. Displacement of the disk can usually be readily identified (Abolmaali et al., 2004; Babadag et al., 2004). Investigators have reported in patients with disk displacement without reduction that MRI generally reveals greater tissue change and joint effusion on T2-weighted images than those patients with reduction (Sener and Akgunlu, 2003; Yamamoto et al., 2003) (Figures 3–41 to 3–44).

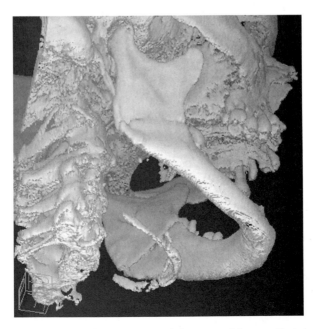

Figure 3–40 This three-dimensional CT image reveals fractures of the mandibular angles bilaterally.

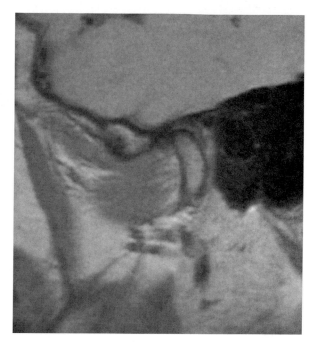

Figure 3–41 In this sagittal MRI of a 36-year old female, the disk on the asymptomatic right is positioned normally in the fossa superior to the mandibular condyle.

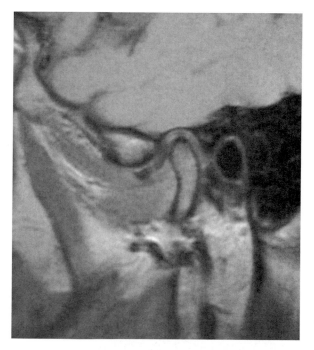

Figure 3–42 On the symptomatic left during closure, note the anterior position of the disk in comparison to the asymptomatic side.

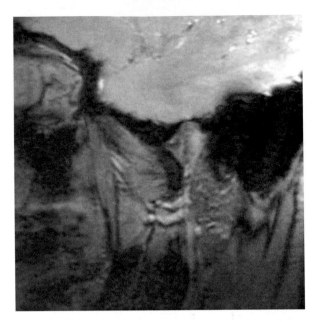

Figure 3–43 In this image, captured during opening movement, the disk on the asymptomatic right is properly positioned between the mandibular condyle and articular eminence.

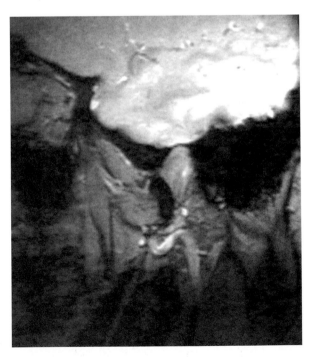

Figure 3–44 This image on the symptomatic left, also captured during opening movement, reveals a forwardly displaced disk which is folding and kinking. The findings of the images are consistent with disk displacement without reduction.

MRI is capable of demonstrating bony changes on T1-weighted images, including changes as severe as arthrosis to more subtle anomalies such as marrow edema (Emshoff et al., 2003c; Brandlmaier et al., 2003). Osteoarthrosis of the joint is most readily demonstrated on T1-weighted images by flattening of the condyle, sclerosis, surface irregularities, and possibly erosion (Emshoff et al., 2003c; Yura and Totsuka, 2005). Marrow edema is suggested by the presence of a hypointense signal on T1- weighted images and increased signal intensity on T2-weighted images. Joint effusion and synovial activity are best demonstrated on T2-weighted images by hyperintense signal (Emshoff et al., 2003c; Yura and Totsuka, 2005).

As an alternative to MRI due to expense and patient claustrophobia, the use of ultrasound to image the joint has recently been investigated. Ultrasonography has been reported to detect joint effusion with accuracy (Manfredini et al., 2004; Melchiorre et al., 2003). Results of the ability of ultrasound to assess condylar morphology have been inconsistent (Brandlmaier et al., 2003c; Emshoff et al., 2003b; Melchiorre et al., 2003). The sensitivity and specificity of ultrasonography is, however, inferior to MRI in the detection of TMJ internal derangement (Brandlmaier et al., 2003a, 2003c). Among patients with whom MRI is particularly difficult, use of diagnostic ultrasound may be an option, but advancement of the technology must occur before it becomes the first line of imaging for most patients.

CLINICAL RELEVANCE TO PHYSICAL THERAPY

Rehabilitation Implications 1

For patients presenting with spine pain and with diagnosed rheumatoid arthritis or advanced degenerative changes, physical therapists are required to be particularly vigilant in observing for any indication of neurological compromise. In patients with rheumatoid arthritis, the risk of upper cervical instability warrants particular concern as the potential consequences are devastating. Patients with advanced degenerative changes also require specific scrutiny due to the possibility of spinal cord compression due to central canal stenosis. Any indication of neurological compromise demands immediate physician consultation for further medical evaluation. Clinicians are prudent to observe for any indication of neurological disturbance including hyperreflexia, upgoing plantar responses, objective muscle weakness, gait disturbances, myoclonus, Romberg's sign, spasticity, and bowel and bladder control issues.

Rehabilitation Implications 2

Physical therapists regularly provide care for patients with traumatic cervical spine injuries, often with onset in motor vehicle accidents or other high-energy trauma. Adequate viewing of all the potentially injured structures of the cervical spine is not easily managed by the radiologist in cervical spine radiographs. The overlap of bony structures complicates the assessment of tissue integrity, even with multiple views. Certain upper cervical lesions can only be safely ruled out with more detailed imaging such as that offered by CT. The odontoid process, atlas, and occipital condyles frequently require visualization by CT for a thorough investigation confidently ruling out fracture. Failure to identify such an injury potentially leads to catastrophic results. While radiography is usually adequate, use of CT is growing to rule out some occasionally elusive injuries. Use of CT for the cervical spine is mandated following trauma in the presence of conditions predisposing for fracture, such as ankylosing spondylitis.

ADDITIONAL READING

El-Khoury, GY, Kathol, MH., & Daniel, WW. (1995). Imaging of acute injuries of the cervical spine: value of plain radiography, CT., and MR imaging. *American Journal of Roentgenology, 164,* 43–50.

Flanders, A.E., Spettell, C. M., Tartaglino, L.M., et al. (1996). Forecasting motor recovery after cervical spinal cord injury: value of MR imaging. *Radiolgy, 2001,* 649–655.

Ingle, G., Sastre-Garriga, J., Miller, D., & Thompson, A. (2005). Is inflammation important in early PPMS? *Journal of Neurology, Neurosurgery, and Psychiatry, 76,* 1255–1258.

Melhem, ER., Benson, ML., & Beauchamp, NJ. (1996). Cervical spondylosis: three dimensional gradient echo MR with magnetization transfer. *American Journal of Neuroradiology, 17,* 705–711.

Monsey, R. (1997). Rheumatoid arthritis of the cervical spine. *Journal of Academy of Orthopedic Surgery, 5,* 240–248.

Ross, J. S. (1995). Three dimensional magnetic resonance techniques for the evaluation of cervical degenerative disease. *Neuroimaging Clinics of North America, 5,* 329–348.

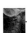

REFERENCES

Cervical Spine

Anderson, L., & D'Alonzo, R. (1974). Fractures of the odontoid process of the axis. *Journal of Bone and Joint Surgery (American), 56,* 1663–1691.

Anderson, P., & Montesano, P. (1988). Morphology and treatment of occipital condyle fractures. *Spine, 13,* 731–736.

Andreshak, J., & Dekutoski, M. (1997). Management of unilateral facet dislocations: a review of the literature. *Orthopedics, 20,* 917–926.

Arnold, D., & Matthews, P. (2003). MRI in the diagnosis and management of multiple sclerosis. *Neurology, 58,* S23–31.

Berlin, L. (2003) CT versus radiography for initial evaluation of cervical spine trauma: what is the standard of care? *American Journal of Radiology, 180,* 911–915.

Boden, S. (1994). Rheumatoid arthritis of the cervical spine: surgical decision making based on predictors of paralysis and recovery. *Spine, 19,* 2275–2280.

Boden, S., Dodge, L., Bohlman, H., & Rechtine, G. (1993). Rheumatoid arthritis of the cervical spine: a long-term analysis with predictors of paralysis and recovery. *Journal of Bone and Joint Surgery (American), 75,* 1282–1297.

Boden, S., McCowin, P., Davis, D., et al. (1990). Abnormal magnetic resonance scans of the cervical spine in asymptomatic subjects. A prospective investigation. *Journal of Bone and Joint Surgery (American), 72,* 1178–1184.

Bogduk, N. (2002). Point of view. *Spine, 27,* 1895.

Borchgrevink, G., Smevik, O, Haave, I., et al. (1997). MRI of the cerebellum and cervical column within two days after whiplash neck sprain injury. *Injury, 28,* 331–335.

Capunao, C., Costagliola, C., Shamsaldin, M., Maleci, A., & Di Lorenzo, N. (2004). Occipital condyle fractures: a hidden nosologic entity. An experience with 10 cases. *Acta Neuroschier (Wien).* 146:779–84.

Cassar-Pullicino, V. (1999). The spine in rheumatologic disorders. *Imaging, 11,* 104–118.

Chamberlain, W. (1939). Basilar impression (platybasia). A bizarre developmental anomaly of the occipital bone and upper cervical spine with striking and misleading manifestations. *Yale Journal of Biology and Medicine, 11,* 487–496.

Chan, S., Shungdu, D., Douglas-Akinwande, A., et al. (1999). Motor neuron diseases: comparison of single-voxel proton MR spectroscopy of the motor cortex with MR imaging of the brain. *Radiology, 212,* 763–769.

Chen, C., Hsu, H., Niu, C., et al. (2003). Cervical degenerative disease at flexion-extension MR imaging: predicion criteria. *Radiology, 227,* 136–142.

Chin, C. (2003). Spine imaging. *Seminars in Neurology, 22,* 205–220.

Clark, C., Goetz , D., & Menezes, A. (1989). Arthrodesis of the cervical spine in rheumatoid patients. *Journal of Bone and Joint Surgery (American), 71,* 381–392.

Collins, D., Barne, S., & Fitzrandolph, R. (1991). Cervical spine instability in rheumatoid patients having total hip or total knee arthroplasty. *Clinical Orthopaedics and Related Research, 272,* 127–135.

Daffner, R. (2001). Helical CT of the cervical spine for trauma patients: a time study. *American Journal of Roentgenology, 177,* 677–679.

Dellestable, F., & Gaucher, A. (1998). Clay shoveler's fracture. Stress fracture of the lower cervical and upper thoracic spinous processes. *Revue du Rhumatisme. English Edition, 65,* 575–582.

Effendi, B., Roy, D., Cornish, B., et al. (1981). Fractures of the ring of the atlas. A classification based on analysis of 131 cases. *Journal of Bone and Joint Surgery (British), 63,* 319–327.

Ernst, C., Stadnik, T., Peeters, E., et al. (2005). Prevalence of annular tears and disc herniations on MR images of the cervical spine in symptom free volunteers. *European Journal of Radiology, 55,* 409–414.

Fujimura, Y, Nishi, Y, & Kobayashi, K. (1996). Classification and treatment of axis body fractures. *Jorurnal of Orthopaedic Trauma, 10,* 536–540.

Fujiwara, K., Fujimoto, M., Owaki, H., et al. (1998). Cervical lesions related to the systemic progression in rheumatoid arthritis. *Spine, 23,* 2052–2056.

Grabb, P., & Pang, D. (1994). Magnetic resonance imaging in the evaluation of spinal cord injury without radiographic abnormality. *Neurosurgery, 1994,* 406–414.

Goldberg, W., Mueller, C., Panacek, E., et al. (2001). NEXUS Group. Distribution patterns of blunt traumatic cervical spine injury. *Annals of Emergency Medicine, 38,* 17–21.

Gore, D. (2001). Roentgenographic findings in the cervical spine in asymptomatic persons: a ten-year follow-up. *Spine, 26,* 2463–2466.

Greenspan, A. (2000). *Orthopedic radiology.* 3rd ed. Philadelphia: Lippincott Williams and Wilkins.

Grogan, E., Morris, J., Dittus, R., et al. (2005). Cervical spine evaluation in urban trauma centers: lowering institutional costs and complications through helical CT scan. *Journal of the American College of Physicians, 200,* 160–165.

Grubb, S., & Kelly, C. (2000). Cervical discography: clinical implications from 12 years of experience. *Spine, 25,* 1382–1389.

Gurley, J., Bell, G. (1997). Surgical management of patients with rheumatoid cervical spine disease. *Rheumatic Disease Clinics of North America, 23,* 317–332.

Guyer, R., Ohnmeiss, D., Mason, S., & Shelokov, A. (1997). Complications of cervical discography: findings in a large series. *Journal of Spinal Disorders, 10,* 95–101.

Haidar, S., Drake, J., & Armstrong, D. (2005). Cervical ankylosis following Grisel's syndrome in a 14-year old boy with infectious mononucleosis. *Pediatric Radiology, 35,* 330–333.

Hanson, J., Blackmore, C., Mann, F., & Wilson, A. (2000). Cervical spine injury. A clinical decision rule to identify high-risk patients for helical CT screening. *American Journal of Roentgenology, 174,* 713–718.

Hanson, J., Deliganis, A., Baxter, A., et al. (2002). Radiologic and clinical spectrum of occipital condyle fractures: retrospective review of 107 consecutive fractures in 95 patients. *American Journal of Roentgenology, 178,* 1261–1268.

Harris, J. (2001). Cervicocranium: its radiographic assessment. *Radiology, 218,* :337–351.

Hayashi, K., Yone, K., Ito, H., et al. (1995). MRI findings in patients with cervical spinal cord injury who do not show radiographic evidence of a fracture or dislocation. *Paraplegia, 33,* 212–215.

Heffez, D., Ros, R., Shade-Zeldow, Y, et al. (2004). Clinical evidence for cervical myelopathy due to Chiari malformation and spinal stenosis in a non-randomized group of patients with the diagnosis of fibromyalgia. *European Spine Journal, 13,* 516–523.

Holmes, J., & Akkinepalli, R. (2005). Computed tomography versus plain radiography to screen for cervical spine injury: a meta-analysis. *Journal of Trauma, 58,* 902–905.

Hopkinson, N, Stevenson, J., & Benjamin, S. (2001). A case ascertainment study of septic discitis: clinical, microbiological and radiological features. *Quarterly Journal of Medicine, 94,* 465–470.

Imhof, H., Fuchsjäger M. (2002). Traumatic injuries: imaging of spinal injuries. *European radiology,* 12, 1262–72.

Jarolimek, A., Coffey, E., Sandler, C., & West, O. (2004). Imaging of upper cervical spine injuries—part III: C2 below the dens. *Applied Radiology, 33,* 9–21.

Kaale, B., Krakenes, J., Albrektsen, G., & Wester, K. (2005). Whiplash-associated disorders impairment rating: neck disability index score according to severity of MRI findings of ligaments and membranes in the upper cervical spine. *Journal of Neurotrauma, 22,* 466–475.

Kaiser, JA., & Holland, BA. (1998). Imaging of the cervical spine. *Spine,* 23, 2701–12.

Kalita, M., Shah, S., Kapoor, R., & Misra, U. (2002). Bladder dysfunction in acute transverse myelitis: magnetic resonance imaging and neurophysiological and urodynamic correlations. *Journal of Neurology, Neurosurgery and Psychiatry, 73,* 154–159.

Karagianis, A., Klufas, R., & Schwartz, R. (2003). MRI of cervical neoplasms. *Applied Radiology Dec,32,* 26–38.

Karlsborg, M., Smed, A., Jespersen, H., et al. (1997). A prospective study of 39 patients with whiplash injury. *Acta Neurologica Scandinavica 95,* 65–72.

Kauppi, M., & Neva, M. (1998). Sensitivity of lateral view cervical spine radiographs taken in the neutral position in atlanto-axial subluxation in rheumatic diseases. *Clinical Rheumatology, 17,* 511–514.

Kauppi, M., Sakaguchi, M., Konttinen, Y., & Hamalainen, M. (1990). A new method of screening for vertical atlantoaxial dislocation., *Journal of Rheumatology 17,* 167–172.

Khanna, A., Carbone, J., Kebiash,K., et al. (2002). Magnetic resonance imaging of the cervical spine. *Journal of Bone and Joint Surgery (American), 84,* S70–80.

Kolen, E., & Schmidt, M. (2002). Rheumatoid arthritis of the cervical spine. *Seminars in Urology, 22,* 179–186.

Kopacz, K., & Connolly, P. (1999). The prevalence of cervical spondylolisthesis. *Orthopedics, 22,* 677–679.

Krakenes, J., Kaale, B., Moen, G., et al. (2003). MRI of the tectorial and posterior atlanto-occipital membranes in the late stage of whiplash injury. *Neuroradiolgy, 45,* 585–591.

Krakenes, J., Kaale, B., Moen, G., et al. (2002). MRI of the alar ligaments in the late stage of whiplash injury—a study of structural abnormalities and observer agreement. *Neuroradiology, 44,* 617–624.

Kwan, O. (2003). MRI assessment of the alar ligaments in the late stage of whiplash injury. *Neuroradiology, 45,*195–196.

Leone, A., Cerase, A., Colosimo, C., et al. (2000). Occipital condylar fractures: a review. *Radiology, 216,* 635–644.

Lewis, L., Docherty, M., Ruoff, B., et al. (2001). Flexion-extension views in the evaluation of cervical spine injuries. *Annals of Emergency Medicine, 20,* 117–121.

Lingawi, S. (2001). The naked facet sign. *Radiology, 219,* 366–367.

Lomoschitz, F., Blackmore, C., Mirza, S., & Mann, F. (2002). Cervical spine injuries in patients 65 years old and older: epidemiologic analysis regarding the effects of age and injury mechanism on distribution, type, and stability of injuries. *American Journal of Roentgenology, 178,* 573–577.

Loughrey, G., Collins, C., Todd, S., et al. (2000). Magnetic resonance imaging in the management of suspected spinal canal disease in patients with known malignancy. *Clinical Radiology, 55,* 849–855.

McGregor, M. (1948). The significance of certain measurements of the skull in the diagnosis of basilar impression. *British Journal of Radiology, 21,* 171–181.

McRae, D., & Barnum, A. (1953). Occipitalization of the atlas. *American Journal of Roentgenology, 70,* 23–45.

Maiuri, F., Iaconetta, G., Gallicchio, B., et al. (1997). Spondylodiscitis: clinical and magnetic resonance diagnosis. *Spine, 22,* 1741–1746.

Manaster, B., & May, D. (2002). Spine trauma. In, Manaster. B. J., Disler, D. G., May, D. A. (eds.). *Musculoskeletal imaging. The requisites.* 2nd ed. St. Louis: Mosby.

Matar, L., Helms, C., & Richardson, W. (2003). Spinolaminar breach: an important sign in cervical spinous process fractures. *Skeletal Radiology, 29,* 75–80.

Matsumoto, M., Fujimura, Y, Suzdki, N. (1998). MR of cervical intervertebral disks in asymptomatic subjects. *Journal of Bone and Joint Surgery (British), 80,* 19–24.

Maus, T. (2002). Imaging of the spine and nerve roots. *Physical Medicine and Rehabilitation Clinics of North America, 13,* 487–544.

Mehdorn, H., Fritsch ,M., & Stiller, R. (2005). Treatment options and results in cervical myelopathy. *Acta Neurochirugica Supplement (Wien), 93,*177–182.

Mintz, DN. (2004). Magnetic resonance imaging of sports injuries to the cervical spine. *Seminars in Musculoskeletal Radiology, 8,* 99–110.

Muhle,C., Metzner, J., Weinert, D., et al. (1998). Classification system based on kinematic MR imaging in cervical spondylitic myelopathy. *American Journal of Neuroradiology, 19,* 1763–1771.

Müller, EJ., Wick, M., Russe, O., & Muhr, G. (1999). Management of odontoid fractures in the elderly. *European Spine Journal, 8,* 360–365.

Nakstad, P., Server, A., & Josefsen, R. (2004). Traumatic cervical injuries in ankylosing spondylitis. *Acta Radiologica, 45,* 222–226.

Nguyen, G., & Clark, R. (2005). Adequacy of plain radiography in the diagnosis of cervical spine injuries. *Emergency Radiology, 11,* 158–161.

Okada, Y, Fukasawa, N, Tomomasa, T., et al. (2002). Atlanto-axial subluxation (Grisel's syndrome) associated with mumps. *Pediatrics International, 44,* 192–194.

Okada, Y, Ikada, T., Sakamoto, R., et al. (1993). Magnetic resonance imaging study on the results of surgery for cervical compression myelopathy. *Spine, 23,* 2052–2056.

Papadopoulos, S., Seldon, N, Quint, D., & Patel, N. (2002). Immediate spinal cord decompression for cervical spinal cord injury: feasibility and outcome. *Journal of Trauma, 52,* 323–332.

Pape, E. (2004).Comments on MRI of the tectorial and posterior atlanto-occipital membranes in the late stage of whiplash injury. *Neuroradiology, 46,* 84–485.

Parfenchuck, T., & Janssen, M. (1994). A correlation of cervical magnetic resonance imaging and discography/computed tomographic discograms. *Spine, 19,* 2819–2825.

Pathria, M. (2005). Imaging of spine instability. *Seminars in Musculoskeletal Radiology, 9,* 88–99.

Pedrosa, I, Jorquera, M., Mendez, R., Cabeza, B.(2002). Cervical spine fractures in ankylosing spondylosis: MR findings. *Emergency Radiology, 9,* 38–42.

Pellei, D. (2000). The fat C2 sign. *Radiology, 215,* 359–360.

Perronne, C., Saba, J., Behloul, Z, et al. (1994). Pyogenic and tuberculous spondylodiscitis (vertebral osteomyelitis) in 80 adult patients. *Clinical Infectious Diseases, 19,* 746–750.

Pollack, C., Hendey, G., Martin, D., Hoffman, J., & Mower, W. Nexus Group. (2002). Use of flexion-extension radiographs of the cervical spine in blunt trauma. *Annals Emergency Medicine, 38,* 8–11.

Ranawat, C., O'Leary, P., Pellicci, P., et al. (1979). Cervical spine fusion in rheumatoid arthritis. *Journal of Bone and Joint Surgery (American), 61,* 1003–1010.

Redla, S., Sikdar, T., Saifaddin, A., & Taylor B. (1999). Imaging features of cervical spondylosis with emphasis on MR appearances. *Clinical Radiology, 54,* 815–820.

Redlund-Johnell, I, & Pettersson, H. (1984). Radiographic measurements of the cranio-vertebral region. Designed for evaluation of abnormalities in rheumatoid arthritis. *Acta Radiologica Diagnostica (Stockholm), 25,* 23–28.

Reijnierse M., Dijkmans B., Hansen B., et al. (2001). Neurologic dysfunction in patients with rheumatoid arthritis of the cervical spine. Predictive value of clinical, radiographic, and MR imaging parameters. *European Radiology, 11,* 467–473.

Richards, P. (2005). Cervical spine clearance: a review. *Injury, 36,* 248–269.

Riew, D., Hilibrand, A., Palumbo, M., et al. (2001). Diagnosing basilar invagination in the rheumatoid patient: the reliability of radiographic data. *Journal of Bone and Joint Surgery (American), 83,* 194–200.

Roche, C., Eyes, B., & Whitehouse, G. The rheumatoid cervical spine: signs of instability on plain cervical radiographs. *Clinical Radiology, 57,* 241–249.

Roh, J., Teng, A., Yoo, J., et al. (2005). Degenerative disorders of the lumbar and cervical spine. *Orthopedic Clinics of North America, 36,* 255–262.

Ronnen, H., Korte, P., Brink, P., et al. (1996). Acute whiplash injury: is there a role for MRI? A prospective study of 100 patients. *Radiology, 201,* 93–96.

Rothman, SLG. (1996). The diagnosis of infections of the spine by modern imaging techniques. *Orthopedic Clinics of North America, 27,* 15–31.

Schellhas, K., Garvey, T., Johnson, B., et al., (2003). Cervical diskography: analysis of provoked responses at C2-C3, C3-C4, and C4-C5. *American Journal of Neuroradiology, 21,* 269–275.

Schellhas, K., Smith, M., Gundry, C., & Pollei, S. (1996). Cervical discogenic pain. Prospective correlation of magnetic resonance imaging and discography in asymptomatic subjects and pain sufferers. *Spine, 21,* 300–311.

Shanmuganathan, K., Mirvis, S., Dowe, M., & Levine, A. (1996). Traumatic isolation of the cervical articular pillar: imaging observations in 21 patients. *American Journal of Roentgenology, 166,* 897–902.

Siivola, S., Levoska, S., Tervonen, O., et al. (2002). MRI changes of cervical spine in asymptomatic and symptomatic young adults. *European Spine Journal, 11,* 358–363.

Slipman, C., Plastaras, C., Patel, R., et al. (2005). Provocative cervical discography symptom mapping. *Spine Journal, 5,* 381–388.

Stafira, J., Sonnad ,J., Yuh ,W., et al. (2003). Qualitative assessment of cervical stenosis: observer variability on CT and MR images. *American Journal of Neuroradiology, 24,* 766–769.

Stark, D., & Bradley, W. (1999). *Magnetic resonance imaging.* 3rd ed. Vol. 3. St. Louis: Mosby.

Steill, I, Wells, G., Vandemheen, K., et al. (2001). The Canadian C-spine rule for radiography in alert and stable trauma patients. *JAMA, 286,* 1841–1848.

Steinberg, E., Ovadia, D., Nissan, M., et al. (2005). Whiplash injury: is there a role for electromyographic studies? *Archives of Orthopaedic and Trauma Surgery, 125,* 46–50.

Stosic-Opincal, T., Peric, V., Grujicic, D., et al. (2004). The role of magnetic resonance imaging in the diagnosis of post-operative spondylodiscitis. *Vojnosanit Pregl, 61,* 479–483.

Suda,K., Abumi, K., Ito, M., et al. (2003). Local kyphosis reduces surgical outcomes of expansive open-door laminoplasty for cervical spondylotic myelopathy. *Spine, 28,* 1258–1262.

Swischuk, L. (1999). Normal cervical spine variations mimicking injuries in children. *Emergency Radiology, 1,* 299–306.

Tali, E. (2004). Spinal infections. *European Journal of Radiology, 50,*120–133.

Teresi, L., Lufkin, R., & Reicher, M. (1987). Asymptomatic degenerative disk disease and spondylosis of the cervical spine. *Radiology, 164,* 83–88.

Tewari, M., Gifti, D., Singh, P., et al. (2005). Diagnosis and prognostication of adult spinal cord injury without radiographic abnormality using magnetic resonance imaging: analysis of 40 patients. *Surgical Neurology, 63,* 204–209.

Transverse myelitis consortium working group (2002). Proposed diagnostic criteria and nosology of acute transverse myelitis. *Neurology, 59,* 499–505.

Tuli, S., Tator, C., Fehlings, M., & Mackay, M. (1997). Occipital condyle fractures. *Neurosurgery, 41,* 368–376.

Vandemark, R. (1990). Radiology of the cervical spine in trauma patients: practice pitfalls and recommendations for improving efficiency and communications. *American Journal of Roentgenology, 155,* 155:465–472.

Van Goethem, J., Maes, M., Ozsarlak, O., et al. (2005). Imaging in spinal trauma. *European Radiology, 15,* 582–590.

Voyvodic, F., Dolinis, J., Moore, V., et al. (1997). MRI of car occupants with whiplash injury. *Neuroradiology, 39,* 35–40.

Wackenhelm, A. (1974). *Roentgen diagnosis of the cranio-vertebral region.* New York: Springer.

West, O. (2002). Imaging of upper cervical spine injuries-part I:CO-C1. *Applied Radiology, 31,* 23–32.

West, O, Bilow, R.,& Jaromilek, A. (2003). Imaging of upper cervical spine injuries-part II: the dens. *Applied Radiology, 32,* 30–38.

Widder, S., Doig, C., Burrowes, P., et al. (2004). Prospective evaluation of computed tomographic scanning for spinal clearance of obtunded trauma patients: preliminary results. *Journal of Trauma, 56,* 1179–1184.

Wilmink, J., & Patijn, J. MR imaging of alar ligament in whiplash-associated disorders: an observer study. *Neuroradiology, 43,* 859–863.

Wolfe, B., O'Keefe, D., Mitchell, D., & Tchang, S. (1987).Rheumatoid arthritis of the cervical spine: early and progressive radiographic features. *Radiology, 165,* 145–148.

Yousem, D. M., Atlas, S. W., Goldberg, H. I., & Grossman, R. I. (1991). Degenerative narrowing of the cervical spine neural foramina: evaluation with high-resolution 3-DFT gradient-echo MR Imaging. *American Journal of Radiology, 12,* 229–236.

Zeidman, S., & Ducker, T. (1994). Rheumatoid arthritis: neuroanatomy, compression, and grading deficits. *Spine, 19,* 2259–2266.

Zeidman S., Thompson K., Ducker T. Complications of cervical discography: analysis of 4400 diagnostic disc injections. Neurosurg 1995;37:414–417.

Zheng Y, Liew S., Simmons E. Value of magnetic resonance imaging and discography in determining the level of cervical discectomy and fusion., *Spine,* 2004;29:2140–2145.

Temporomandibular Joint

Abolmaali, N., Schmitt, J., Schwartz, W., et al. (2004). Visualization of the articular disk of the temporomandibular joint in near-real-time MRI: feasibility study. *European Radiology, 14,* 1889–1894.

Babadag, M., Sahin, M., & Gorgun, S. (2004). Pre- and posttreatment analysis of clinical symptoms of patients with temporomandibular disorders. *Quintessence International, 35,* 811–814.

Brandlmaier, I., Bertram, S., Rudisch, A., et al. (2003a). Temporomandibular joint osteoarthrosis diagnosed with high resolution ultrasonography versus magnetic resonance imaging: how reliable is high resolution ultrasonography? *Journal of Oral Rehabilitation, 30,* 812–817.

Brandlmaier, I., Gruner, S., Rudisch, A., et al. (2003b). Validation of the clinical diagnositic criteria for temporomandibular disorders for the diagnostic subgroup of degenerative joint disease. *Journal of Oral Rehabilitation, 30,* 401–406.

Brandlmaier, I., Rudisch , A., Bodner, G., et al. (2003c). Temporomandibular joint internal derangement: detection with 12.5 MHz ultrasonography. *Journal of Oral and Maxillofacial Rehabilitation, 30,* 796–801.

Dias, G., Premachandra, I., Mahoney, P., & Kieser, J. (2005). A new approach to improve TMJ morphological information from plain film radiographs. *Cranio, 23,* 30–38.

Emshoff, R., Brandlmaier, I., Bertram, S., & Rudisch, A. (2003a). Risk factors for temporomandibular joint pain in patients with disc displacement without reduction—a magnetic resonance imaging study. *Journal of Oral and Maxillofacial Rehabilitation, 30,* 537–543.

Emshoff, R., Brandlmaier, I., Bodner, G., & Rudisch, A. (2003b). Condylar erosion and disc displacement: detection with high-resolution ultrasonography. *Journal of Oral and Maxillofacial Surgery, 61,* 877–881.

Emshoff, R., Brandlmaier, I., Schmid, C., et al. (2003c). Bone marrow edema of the mandibular condyle related to internal derangement., osteoarthrosis, and joint effusion. *Journal of Oral and Maxillofacial Rehabilitation, 61,* 35–40.

Gorgu, M., Erdogan, B., Akoz, T., et al. (2000). Three-dimensional computed tomography in evaluation of ankylosis of the temporomandibular joint. *Scandinavian Journal of Plastic Reconstructive Hand Surgery, 34,* 117–120.

Honda, K., Arai, Y, Kashima, M., et al. (2004). Evaluation of the usefulness of the limited cone-beam CT (3DX) in the assessment of the thickness of the roof of the glenoid fossa of the temporomandibular joint. *Dentomaxillofacial Radiology, 33,* 391–395.

Manfredini, D., Tognini, F., Melchiorre, D., et al. (2003). The role of ultrasonography in the diagnosis of temporomandibular joint disc displacement and intra-articular effusion. *Minerva Stomatology, 52,* 52:93–1004.

Melchiorre, D., Calderazzi, A., Bongi, S., et al. (2003). A comparison of ultrasonography and magnetic resonance imaging in the evaluation of temporomandibular joint involvement in rheumatoid arthritis and psoriatic arthritis. *Rheumatology, 42,* 673–676.

Sener, S., & Akgunlu, F. (2004). MRI characteristics of anterior disc displacement with and without reduction. *Dentomaxillofacial Radiology, 33,* 245–252.

Yamamoto, M., Sano, T., & Okano, T. (2003). Magnetic resonance evidence of joint fluid with temporomandibular joint disorders. *Journal of Computer Assisted Tomography, 27,* 694–698.

Yura, S., & Totsuka, Y. (2005). Relationship between effectiveness of athrocentesis under sufficient pressure and conditions of the temporomandibular joint. *Journal of Oral and Maxillofacial Surgery, 63,* 225–228.

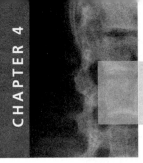

CHAPTER 4

Imaging of the Thoracolumbar Spine

Images of normal anatomy reveal the typical lumbar spine consisting of five lumbar vertebrae, featuring rectangular bodies. From a lateral view or in sagittal slices, the interposed disks increase in height with caudal progression, although the L5–S1 disk is variable (Maus, 2002).

Of principal importance is the general contour of the spine. The curvilinear alignment of the vertebrae is represented on a lateral view or sagittal slices by (Maus, 2002; Savitsky and Votey, 1997; Imhof and Fuchsjäger, 2002) (Figures 4–1 and 4–2):

1. A line spanning the anterior margins of the vertebral bodies: anterior spinal line.

2. A line adjoining the posterior margins of the vertebral bodies: posterior spinal line.

3. The line adjoining the junctions of the laminae and the anterior margins of the spinous processes: spinolaminar line.

4. A line along the tips of the spinous processes: spinous process line.

In axial images, the posterior margins of the disks and vertebral bodies are concave, contributing to a usually triangular spinal canal (Figure 4–3). The posterior aspect of the L5–S1 disk can again be less consistent in its contribution to this form. With caudal progression in the lumbar spine, the interpedicular distance increases (Maus, 2002).

In the thoracic spine, many of the same elements exist as in the lumbar region, including increasing vertebral body size with caudal progression. The intervertebral disks, however, are proportionally smaller within the motion segments. The interpedicular distance decreases from T1 to T6, then increases again through T12 (Maus, 2002).

The ligamentous and neural structures of the thoracic and lumbar spines are demonstrated most clearly on magnetic resonance imaging (MRI). The bony apertures for the neural structures are best seen by computed tomography (CT) or MRI, as are the pars interarticulares and the facet joints (Maus, 2002; Savitsky and Votey, 1997; Imhof and Fuchsjäger, 2002).

The spinal cord in the thoracic region has a round to oval cross section, expanding normally at the conus, the tip of which is usually at L1 or L2. The appearances of the thoracic and lumbar spines on MRI are dependent on age as changes in the marrow of the vertebral bodies occur in adulthood. Similarly, the proportion of nuclear material with the disk reduces with maturity (Maus, 2002).

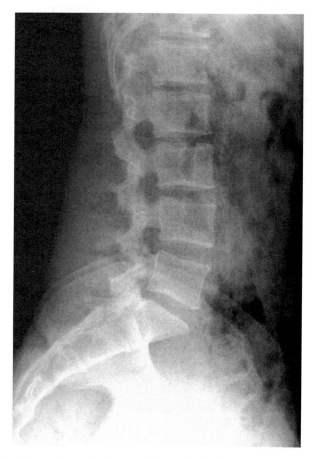

Figure 4–1 A lateral view radiograph of a normal-appearing lumbar spine in a 19-year-old male. Note the alignment of the anterior and posterior vertebral bodies, the spinolaminar line, and the tips of the spinous processes.

On T1-weighted MRI, the cerebrospinal fluid is of low signal intensity in contrast to the intermediate signal from the spinal cord. Osseous structures including the vertebral body, pedicles, laminae, and transverse and spinous processes demonstrate high signal intensity. The intervertebral disk is described by the nucleus pulposus being of intermediate signal and the surrounding annulus fibrosis of lower intensity. On T2-weighted images, the cord is low-intermediate signal and the cerebrospinal fluid is intensely bright. Also on T2-weighted images, the vertebral body is at an intermediate level of intensity. The disks on T2-weighted images demonstrate high signal intensity with the nucleus pulposus and low signal with the annulus fibrosis. The nerve root sleeves are low-intermediate level of signal intensity (Greenspan, 2000) (Figure 4–4).

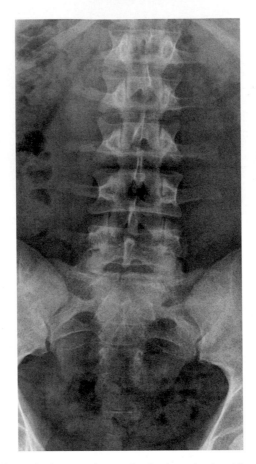

Figure 4–2 An AP radiograph of a normal-appearing lumbar spine in a 19-year-old male.

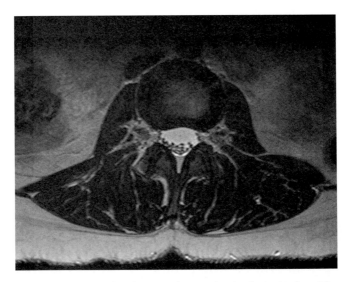

Figure 4–3 T2-weighted axial section of a normal-appearing lumbar spine in a 37-year-old female. Note the triangular spinal canal with ample room for the contained nerve roots.

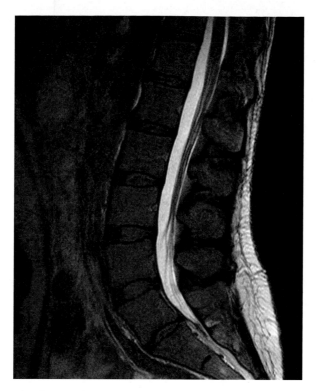

Figure 4–4 T2-weighted image of a normal-appearing lumbar spine in a 35-year-old female. Note the height of the vertebral bodies and disks, the alignment of the vertebral bodies and disk margins, and signal intensity of the disks. Also note the brightness of signal by the CSF surrounding the spinal cord and nerve roots.

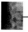 **RADIOGRAPHY**

Radiography remains a valuable entry-level diagnostic study for certain suspected lumbar spine pathologies. The principal advantages of radiography are the low cost and ready availability. The evolution of more sophisticated imaging modalities has, however, reduced the utility of radiography as its levels of sensitivity have been surpassed by CT and MRI for many disorders. The lack of clinically relevant information revealed on radiographs has also been the source of questions more recently examined by investigators. The best utilization of radiography is now perhaps as a screening mechanism and a guide for further imaging (Chin, 2002; Simmons et al., 2003; Khoo et al., 2003; Maus, 2002).

Radiography is now used most frequently for initial investigation of suspected degenerative disorders, spondylolysis, anklyosing spondylitis, metastases (Van den Bosch et al., 2004), and instability (Pitanken et al., 2002).

Initial screening for fractures is also often conducted with radiography, particularly after trauma. Basic skeletal alignment and the integrity of vertebral bodies can be quickly assessed (Chin, 2002). Recent large studies have estimated the sensitivity of lumbar

TABLE 4–1	Three-Column Classification System for the Thoracolumbar Spine		
System	Anterior	Middle	Posterior
Structures	Anterior longitudinal ligament, anterior half of vertebral body, anterior part of annulus fibrosus	Posterior half of vertebral body, posterior longitudinal ligament, posterior part of annulus fibrosus	Pedicles, laminae, ligamentum flavum, facet joint capsules, supraspinous ligament, interspinous ligaments

radiography to detect fractures at 75 percent (Herzog et al., 2004) and 86 percent (Sheridan et al., 2003). The vertebrae of the thoracolumbar junction are most frequently involved, and there is declining frequency with caudal progression (Holmes et al., 2001; Imhof and Fuchsjäger, 2002). Compression and transverse process fractures are the most frequently identified followed by wedge compression and burst fractures (Holmes et al., 2001).

Of foremost importance in emergent radiologic assessment of the thoracolumbar spine is the determination of spinal stability. The concept of spinal stability is based on the security of the neural elements from encroachment and potential damage by the osteoligamentous structures while the spine is under load (White and Panjabi, 1990; Denis, 1983).

A three-column classification system for the thoracolumbar spine is often used in such radiologic assessment (Denis, 1983), with the overall stability of the spine being largely determined by the integrity of the middle column (Table 4–1).

The three-column classification system for the thoracolumbar spine has become the basis for the thoracolumbar spine injury classification system as proposed by McAfee et al. (1983), with fractures being categorized as major or minor (Table 4–2). Generally, minor fractures pose little to no particular threat to the neural structures and are considered stable. Major injuries may include dislocations as well as fractures, with instability being presumed while emergent care is being provided (Savitsky and Votey, 1997).

The minor fractures are isolated injuries to the transverse or spinous processes or the pars interarticulares. With no compromise of the neural elements, spinal stability is not threatened from an emergent care standpoint (Imhof and Fuchsjäger, 2002; Savitsky and Votey, 1997; Vollmer and Gegg, 1997).

TABLE 4–2	Thoracolumbar Spine Injury Classification
Minor Fractures	**Major Fractures/Dislocations**
Transverse process fractures	Wedge compression fractures
Spinous process fractures	Chance fractures
Pars interarticularis fractures	Burst fractures
	Flexion-distraction injuries
	Translational injuries

Derived as data from: McAfee PC, Hansen YA, Fredrickson BE, et al. (1983). The value of computed tomography in thoracolumbar fractures. Journal of Bone and Joint Surgery (American), 65A, 461–473.

Wedge compression fractures typically result from flexion forces. The anterior column is compressed, while the middle column remains intact. Neurologic compromise is unusual unless there is severe vertebral body height loss or multiple adjacent vertebrae are similarly involved (Imhof and Fuchsjäger, 2002; Savitsky and Votey, 1997; Vollmer and Gegg, 1997) (Figure 4–5).

A chance fracture also results from flexion, but the rotational axis for flexion is more anterior than that causing a wedge compression fracture; typically anterior to the anterior longitudinal ligament. Horizontal disruption of the spinous process, lamina, transverse processes, pedicles, and vertebral body occurs. Historically, this type of injury in the thoracolumbar spine was frequently associated with lap belt use exclusive of the shoulder harness in high-speed motor vehicle accidents (Howland et al., 1965; Savitsky and Votey, 1997; Vollmer and Gegg, 1997).

Burst fractures occur as both the anterior and middle columns fail under axial compression force. The posterior vertebral body cortex is disrupted and the spinal cord is at risk of injury from retropulsion of bone fragments into the spinal canal (Imhof and Fuchsjäger, 2002; Savitsky and Votey, 1997; Vollmer and Gegg, 1997; Kifune et al., 1997).

Flexion-distraction injury occurs with flexion with the axis of rotation between the anterior and posterior longitudinal ligaments. There is compressive failure of the anterior column concurrent with distraction failure in the middle and posterior columns, including rupture of the posterior longitudinal ligament. Instability typically results because of the severity of the disruption (Imhof and Fuchsjäger, 2002; Savitsky and Votey, 1997; Vollmer and Gegg, 1997).

Translational injury results from failure of all three columns owing to shear forces. In the majority of cases, the direction of shear is posterior to anterior. Displacement of the spinal column occurs in the transverse plane, frequently compromising the spinal canal

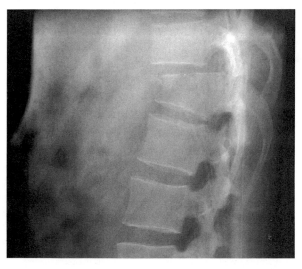

Figure 4–5 Lateral view radiograph demonstrating wedge compression deformity of the T12 vertebral body.

and resulting in neurologic deficit. Instability is the rule with this category of injury, which also includes slice fractures, rotational fracture dislocations, and pure dislocations (Imhof and Fuchsjäger, 2002; Savitsky and Votey, 1997; Vollmer and Gegg, 1997).

Compression fractures typically result from axial loading and may be of traumatic origin or without a particular provocative event. Compression fractures are most common in the elderly in association with osteoporosis, with fracture of the thoracolumbar junction occurring with the greatest frequency (Kifune et al., 1997; Quek, 2002). Most are stable injuries and do not threaten neurologic status, with conservative management being the general rule (Dai et al., 2004). With the loss of vertebral body height from compression, permanent deformity can result, particularly in the thoracic spine more than at the thoracolumbar junction or in the lumbar spine (Cortet et al., 2002). The resultant "dowager's hump" is one of the hallmarks of osteoporosis (Quek, 2002). Radiography is relatively insensitive in detecting early osteoporosis. If osteoporosis is identifiable, however, the common features are increased radiolucency of the vertebra and cortical thinning. Owing to the invagination of the end plates into the weakened vertebral bodies, a so-called "fish" deformity can be evident (Quek, 2002) (Figure 4–6).

Radiography also has limited role in investigating degenerative changes. Features such as disk space narrowing, osteophyte formation along the margins of the disks and

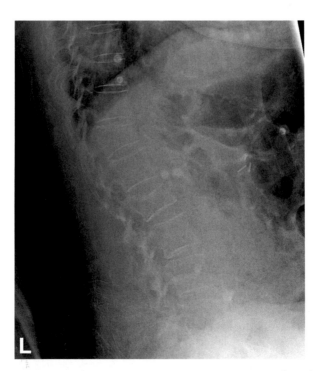

Figure 4–6 A lateral view radiograph in this 75-year-old female reveals significant loss of bone density as the upper lumbar and lower thoracic vertebral bodies are almost radiolucent. Also note the compression fractures present at T12 and L2.

vertebral bodies, and the intradiskal vacuum phenomenon all indicate the progression of significant degenerative disease (Ross, 2000). The vertebral bodies surrounding the affected disks may also demonstrate increased density (Chin, 2002). The difficulty for clinicians recognizing such findings is in determining the applicability of such features relative to the patient's complaints. The presence of degenerative changes in subjects with no history of back pain is well documented, and their presence is only weakly correlated to painful syndromes (Van den Bosch et al., 2004; Peterson et al., 2000; Witt et al., 1984; Torgerson and Dotter, 1976).

While the earliest radiographic changes indicative of ankylosing spondylitis often occur at the sacroiliac joints, several characteristic findings may also be present in the spine. Vertebral body squaring, osteopenia, marginal syndesmophytes, disk calcification, and joint capsule and ligament ossification are indicative of ankylosing spondylitis. Radiographs may also show narrowing circumscribed defects in neighboring vertebral bodies and widening of reactive sclerosis in the surrounding cancellous bone. The disk spaces may become radiolucent with erosions and reactive sclerosis extending into adjacent vertebral bodies (Vinson and Major, 2003). In advanced stages, the characteristic "bamboo spine" may occur as segments fuse and soft tissues become radiopaque (Gran and Skomsvoll, 1997; Sampio-Barros, 2001) (Figure 4–7). In the early phases of the disease, however, radiography is not sensitive to the initial tissue changes (Grigorian et al., 2004; Khan, 2002).

Paget's disease involving the spine is well visualized with radiography. Typical features include coarsening of primary trabeculae, generalized vertebral enlargement, marginal

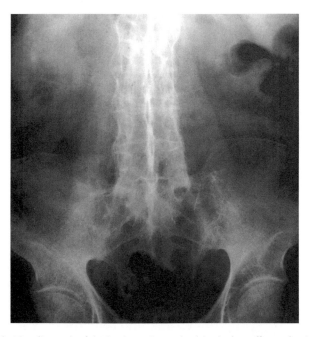

Figure 4–7 In this AP radiograph of the lumbar spine and pelvis, the late effects of ankylosing spondylitis are present. Note the ossification of the intervertebral disks and posterior longitudinal ligament.

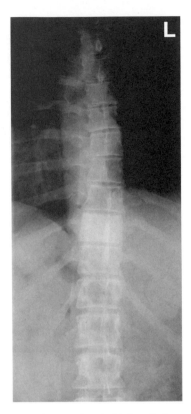

Figure 4–8 The characteristic ivory vertebra associated with Paget's disease is present in this AP radiograph.

sclerosis ("picture frame pattern"), and increased vertebral density involving the neural arch ("ivory vertebrae") (Saiffudin and Hassan, 2003) (Figure 4–8).

Several investigators have proposed limited use of radiography in the management of atraumatic low back pain (Van den Bosch et al., 2004; Simmons et al., 2003; Anderson et al., 2000; Bell and Modic, 1992; Scavone et al., 1981). Growing evidence such as a recent analysis of 2100 radiographs of patients with primary complaints of low back pain (Van den Bosch et al., 2004) failed to yield benefit in the inclusion of radiography as a diagnostic tool. The presence of findings consistent with degenerative changes predictably increased with age, but did not necessarily reveal any information relevant to intervention. In this study, the probability of detecting cancer or infection was determined to be 1 in 1000. Thus, identifying serious pathology on radiographs is a remote possibility. Further, with the probability that radiographically occult soft tissue injury is the likely symptom of origin in the atraumatic onset of low back pain, there is little rationale to include radiography in the overall management of the typical patient presenting with low back pain. Similarly, the association between anatomic variants and the development of back pain has been reported inconsistently (Steinberg et al., 2003; Witt et al., 1984) (Figure 4–9).

Spondylolysis is reported as occurring in 3 to 6 percent of the population, with the identification often incidental owing to the lumbosacral region typically being asymptomatic

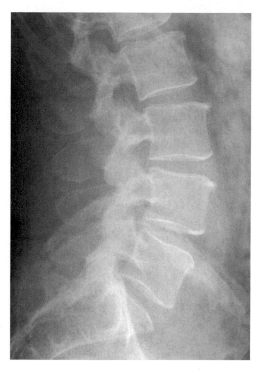

Figure 4–9 In this lateral view radiograph, mild osteophytic lipping is noted along the anterior vertebral body margins. These are typical changes expected in a 40-year-old male.

(Wimberly, 2002; Rossi and Dragoni, 2001). In comparing those with histories of low back pain and those denying such a history, common findings of spina bifida occulta, hemilumbarization, sacralization, hemisacralization, Schmorl's nodes, and early degenerative changes have been noted to occur with equal frequency (Steinberg et al., 2003).

The limited applicability of radiographs in atraumatic low back pain does not hold true in the decision making of pediatric and adolescent patients. In young athletes, radiography is still frequently used for investigation of spondylolysis or spondylolisthesis. While the lack of clinically relevant information is often problematic in interpreting radiographic results in the skeletally mature spine, positive findings have a much higher probability of relevance in the clinical presentations in pediatric and adolescent patients. A recent large study of athletes (Rossi and Dragoni, 2001) presenting with complaints of low back pain found a 13.9 percent frequency of spondylolysis among 4,243 athletes undergoing plain radiography. Of these with such positive findings, a further 47.5 percent had significant slippage to be classified as spondylolisthesis. These investigators reported that such pars defects on radiographs are best revealed with 45-degree oblique and 20-degree cephalad angulation of the beam. The presence of the collar on the "scotty dog" (also "scottie dog") has long been considered pathognomonic (Wimberly, 2002) (Figures 4–10A & B). Due to concerns of gonadal radiation exposure, particularly in adolescence, this view is now infrequent.

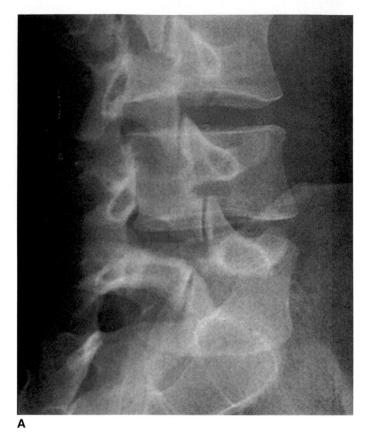

A

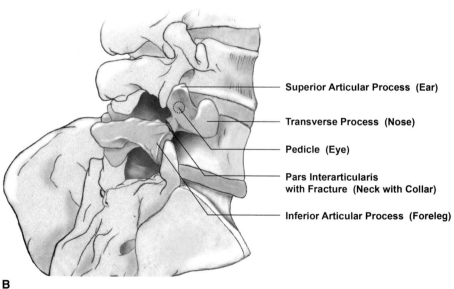

Superior Articular Process (Ear)

Transverse Process (Nose)

Pedicle (Eye)

Pars Interarticularis
with Fracture (Neck with Collar)

Inferior Articular Process (Foreleg)

B

Figure 4–10 A. This posterior oblique view of the lower lumbar spine reveals the "scotty dog" with the collar of increased radiolucency consistent with a fracture of the pars interarticularis. Obtaining this view has fallen out of favor due to concerns of radiation exposure. **B.** The analogous skeletal structures of the "scotty dog" are illustrated. *Illustration courtesy of Tom Dolan, University of Kentucky, Lexington.*

The collar actually demonstrates the pars interarticularis inferior to the pedicle (eye), transverse process (nose), and superior articular process (ear). Projecting from the lamina and spinous process (body) are the inferior articular process (foreleg), the contralateral superior articular process (tail), and contralateral inferior articular process (hindleg) (Greenspan, 2000). Typically, the degree of slippage with spondylolisthesis is categorized by the Taillard (Taillard, 1976) system by citing the percentage of slippage of the superior vertebra over the inferior vertebra or the Meyerding (Meyerding, 1932) grading system, which simply categorizes the percentage of slippage. Grade I reflects up to 25 percent of slippage, while Grade II is 26 to 50 percent, grade III is 51 to 75 percent, grade IV is 76 to 100 percent, and grade V is greater than 100 percent (Wimberly, 2002). Grade V is also known as spondyloptosis (Curylo et al., 2002) (Figures 4–11 and 4–12).

A disorder common in adolescents is Scheuermann's disease, or juvenile kyphosis (Kalifa et al., 2002). The main radiologic sign is disk space narrowing, with anterior involvement being the greatest (Swischuk et al., 1998; Kalifa et al., 2002). This is typically evident between T3–T12, with at least three levels being involved as criteria for the diagnosis of Scheuermann's disease to be applied (Kalifa et al., 2002). (Figure 4–13A & B)

Scoliosis continues to be routinely assessed by radiography with the quantification of the curvature in the coronal plane by the measurement of the Cobb angle (Schwab et al., 2005; Cassar-Pullicino, 2002; Shea et al., 1998). The Cobb angle is measured by

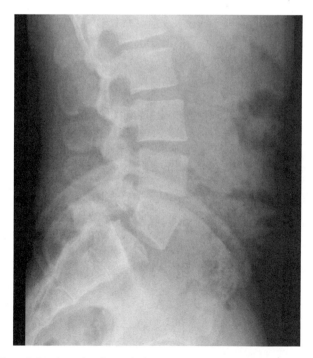

Figure 4–11 A lateral view lateral radiograph demonstrating a grade I spondylolisthesis of L5 on S1. The displacement is perhaps most easily appreciated by the alignment of the posterior margins of the vertebral bodies.

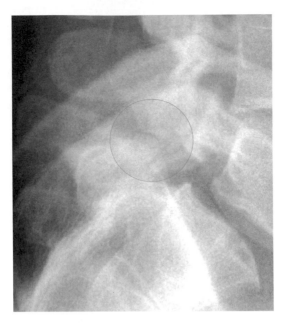

Figure 4–12 Enlargement of the posterior elements of the aforementioned spondylolisthesis image reveals a defect of the pars interarticularis of L5.

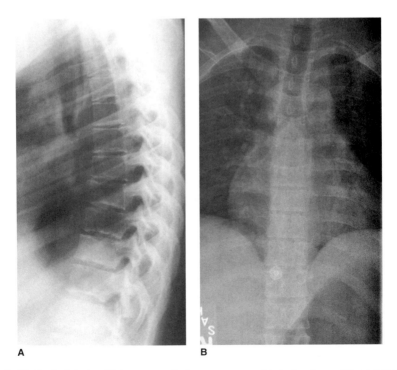

A   B

Figure 4–13 The hallmarks of Scheuermann's disease are present in boths views of these radiographs. Sclerotic changes at the cartilaginous end plate and vertebral body interface and loss of height of the intervertebral disks anteriorly are evident.

identifying the superior and inferior vertebrae of the concavity and drawing lines through their cranial and caudal end plates, respectively. Perpendicular lines are then drawn to intersect from the preceding two lines. The measurement of the intersecting perpendicular lines provides for the Cobb angle (Adam et al., 2005) (Figure 4–14).

Related to the management of scoliosis is the Risser Index, which is a function of ossification of the iliac apophysis. The Risser Index is used as an indicator of vertebral growth and is generally regarded to be more reliable in females (Cassar-Pullicino, 2002).

Perhaps the most specialized use of radiography in the lumbar spine is in the completion of images while the patient is positioned in flexion or extension for suspected motion segment instability, which is likely to be of ligamentous and diskal origin. The term *instability* has become inclusive of multiple definitions and in this context differs from that of concern in emergent care as previously discussed. In the nonemergent patient, neural structures may not be directly threatened, but the mechanical deformation

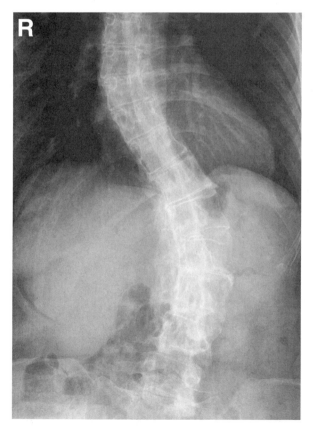

Figure 4–14 An AP radiograph revealing the primary and compensatory curves frequently associated with scoliosis. Note the position of the spinous processes and pedicles indicative of the rotation accompanying the coronal plane deviations.

to the musculoskeletal elements may be the origin of persistent low back pain (Pathria, 2005; Iguchi et al., 2004). Radiologists examine images particularly for translational movement of greater than 4 mm of one vertebra over the subjacent vertebra, abnormal axial rotation of a motion segment, or angular movement of greater than 20 degrees in relation to the adjacent segment (Pitanken, 2002; Maine et al., 2003). In segments demonstrating instability, commensurate degenerative changes have also been reported with variability (Kauppila et al., 1998; Fujiwara et al., 2000; Dupuis et al., 1985).

Radiography is also used to examine the status of cages used in fusion of the lumbar spine. Carbon fiber implants are radiolucent, but recently introduced cages have been equipped with metal markers to allow for ease of examination (Figure 4–15). A fusion is considered successful if (Hanley, 1999; Christensen, 2004):

1. Density is increased or maintained within the cage.
2. No halo or periprosthetic lucency is evident.
3. A sclerotic line between the cage and bone is present suggesting bone formation or remodeling.

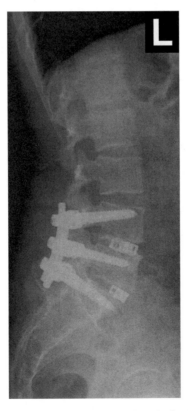

Figure 4–15 A lateral view radiograph exhibiting the posterior spinal rods, pedicle screws, and metallic disk spacers comprising a fusion across L4–S1.

4. Anterior traction spurs undergo resorption or the anterior graft is progressing.

5. No movement is evident on lateral view flexion/extension films.

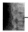

COMPUTED TOMOGRAPHY

CT has consistently demonstrated greater sensitivity and specificity than radiography in imaging bone, particularly in allowing detection and description of fractures. The cortical and trabecular detail of bone can be imaged in remarkable detail, which is particularly of value given the complex anatomy to be considered in the assessment of spine pathology.

The fractures described in the prior section on radiography can, in general, all be more completely represented on CT films than with radiography (Figures 4–16 to 4–18). With the consequences of inaccurate clinical decision making in the immediate care of the patient with a traumatized spine sometimes being devastating, the use of CT has now become routine for many emergency situations, particularly if the patient is unconscious or unable to provide clear subjective report on initial examination (Imhof and Fuchsjäger, 2002; Savitsky and Votey, 1997). The use of CT is valued for the ability to assess for internal organ injury as well as for the osseous structures of the spine (Kuhlman, 1998; Collins, 2000; Herzog, 2004). Use of thin-slice or multiplanar reconstruction can further provide detail well exceeding that of radiography or simple axial CT. An argument can be

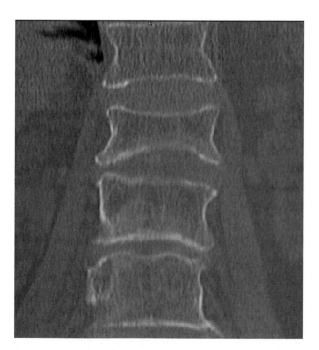

Figure 4–16 Sagittal section of CT soft tissue window view demonstrating obvious osteoligamentous disruption of the thoracic spine.

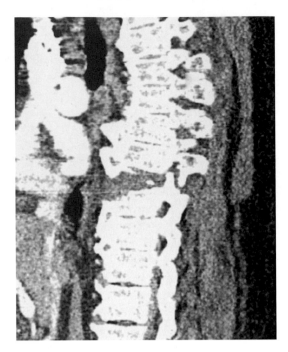

Figure 4–17 Sagittal section of CT soft tissue view demonstrating obvious osteoligamentous disruption of the thoracic spine.

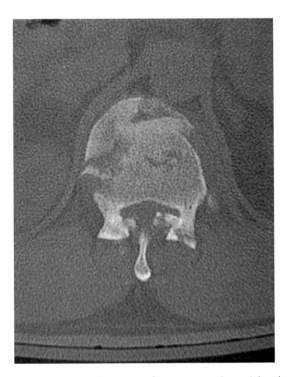

Figure 4–18 Transverse section of CT of T12 burst fracture. Note the peripheral displacement of the fracture fragments.

made for CT being the entry level of imaging for the severely traumatized patient because of higher diagnostic accuracy and cost effectiveness (Bensch et al., 2004).

CT has been suggested to be 25 (Herzog, 2004) to 35 percent (Sheridan, 2003) more sensitive in detection of lumbar spine fractures than radiography, particularly with the addition of multiplanar reconstruction of images. This is especially applicable with subtle fractures of the vertebral bodies and articular processes being revealed with the high signal cortical bone image by CT (Wilmink, 1999). Not only is sensitivity better with CT, but the specificity with which lumbar fractures can be described is greatly improved (Herzog, 2004), particularly with complicated fractures (Arslantas, 2002). Similar data exist for the thoracic spine, with CT demonstrating much greater sensitivity and higher interobserver agreement (Wintermark et al., 2003; Herzog, 2004). The importance of accurate lesion identification and description in clinical decision making is paramount when the risk of neurologic compromise is at issue for the physician managing the patient's emergent care. CT with thin-section or multiplanar reconstruction, therefore, is the preferred imaging modality if a spinal fracture is known or suspected (Jinkins, 2001a).

CT also allows for direct visualization of defects of the pars interarticulares as occurs with spondylolysis and spondylolisthesis (Maus, 2002) and is the best imaging modality for detailing such lesions (Wimberly, 2002). A special application of CT in single-photon emission computed tomography (SPECT) incorporates nuclear imaging and has specific utility for suspect spondylolysis with the greatest sensitivity of any imaging modality and is, thus, the test of choice for diagnosing an occult lesion (Wimberly, 2002). SPECT is capable of detecting the metabolic change at the pars even before standard bone scintigraphy, but is only effective in the acute phase (Rossi and Dragoni, 2001) and has a false-positive rate warranting cautious interpretation (Sys et al., 2001).

While CT is perhaps most recognized for its value in assessment of skeletal integrity, other applications are noteworthy. Owing to its sensitivity in detecting osseous tissue lesions, CT is very effective for allowing examination of the central canal, lateral recesses, and foramina in patients with suspected lumbar spinal stenosis (Maus, 2002; Saifuddin, 2000; Alfieri and Hesselink, 1997). With posterior vertebral body marginal osteophytes and facet hypertrophy typically contributing to the anatomic changes giving rise to stenosis, CT effectively reveals such osseous overgrowth. Several attempts have been made to establish an association between the symptoms of stenosis and specific measurements of these anatomic apertures (Weisz and Lee, 1983; Verbiest, 1977; Bolender et al., 1985), but reliable correlations have yet to be established. MRI reportedly has the tendency to overestimate the degree of stenosis (Taneichi, 2001; Chin, 2002).

CT also readily reveals ossification of ligamentous structures of the lumbar spine as occasionally occurs with the ligamentum flavum and posterior longitudinal ligaments (Hirai, 2001).

CT may also be of value in the diagnosis of tumors of the spine. While soft tissue involvement is best visualized by MRI, CT perhaps best reveals cortical lesions and mineralized matrix abnormalities (Flemming et al., 2000)

The use of CT after myelogram can offer very clinically relevant information that either test in isolation may not reveal. After contrast administration, CT becomes even more sensitive for detecting the anatomic changes associated with stenosis (Saifuddin, 2000;

Taneichi, 2001). The degree of facet arthrosis and subsequent foraminal stenosis are very well defined in post-myelogram CT scans (Ross, 2000). Additionally, bone versus soft tissue intrusion into the foramina may be discriminated by the examiner (Maus, 2002).

Post-myelogram CT in the lumbar spine is generally viewed as having a problem-solving role (Maus, 2002). Such further diagnostic workup may be particularly indicated in patients in whom clinical signs and symptoms do not correlate or in patients who are MRI incompatible (Figures 4–19 to 4–22).

While scoliosis is most noted for the predominant lateral curvature in the coronal plane and often seen adequately with radiography, the deformity is actually three dimensional with altered thoracic kyphosis and rotation often associated with a rib hump on the side of the convexity (Erkula et al., 2003; Cassar-Pullicino, 2002). For extensive involvement, three-dimensional CT may better delineate the deformity (Figure 4–23).

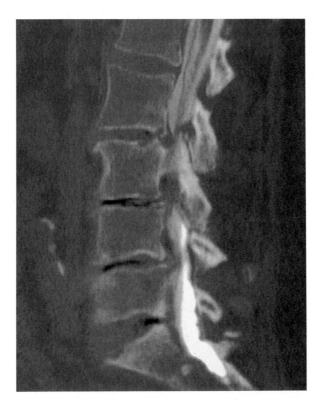

Figure 4–19 This sagittal slice of a post-myelogram CT scan shows severe spinal canal stenosis of congenital and degenerative etiologies. The most severe narrowing, highlighted by the lack of contrast filling the area, is at the L4–5 level.

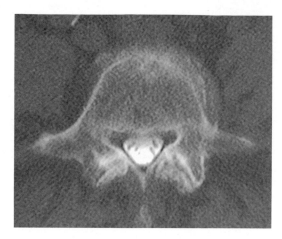

Figure 4–20 This transverse section of the post-myelogram CT scan demonstrates the classic trefoil shape of the spinal canal. Note the congenitally short pedicles and degenerative hypertrophy of the zygapophysial joints.

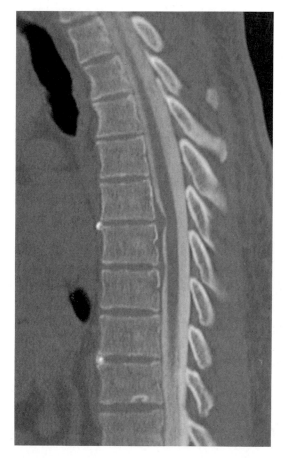

Figure 4–21 A sagittal reconstruction of a post-myelogram CT scan displaying the effacement of the spinal cord due to the protruding thoracic disk. Note the absence of contrast anterior to the spinal cord in the region of the suspected compression.

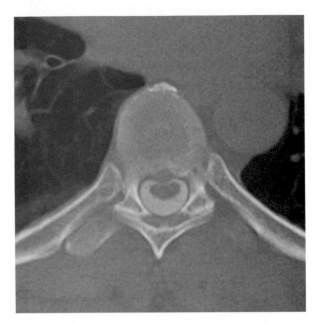

Figure 4–22 An axial section of a post-myelogram CT scan demonstrating a thoracic disk herniation. Note the indentation of the spinal cord due to the protruding disk material.

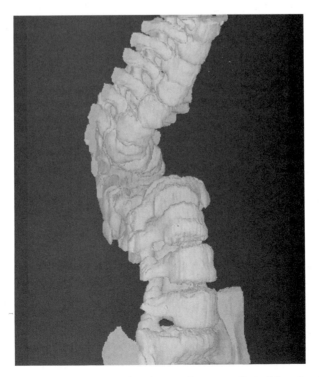

Figure 4–23 An oblique three-dimensional CT image of severe scoliotic deformity of the lower thoracic spine and thoracolumbar junction in an 11-year-old girl.

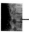
MAGNETIC RESONANCE IMAGING

MRI is the imaging technique of choice for patients with suspected pathologies of soft tissue origin and certain disorders involving the bony elements of the spine. MRI is usually not warranted in the absence of neurologic deficit, a history of trauma, a history of malignancy, or other immunocompromised condition (Taneichi, 2001; Gillan et al., 2001; Fukuda and Kawakami, 2001; Herzog et al., 2004).

T1-weighted images are best for general anatomic orientation because of the bright signal of epidural and foraminal fat. T1-weighted images also depict the bony anatomy relatively well, showing cortical bone as a dark line and cancellous bone as light gray due to the fat content of the marrow (Wilmink, 1999). As such, T1-weighted images are routinely sensitive for images of bone marrow, suspected neoplasm, edema, and reactive degenerative changes (Chin, 2002).

T2-weighted fast spin echo (FSE) images readily reveal the spinal cord, nerve roots, canal size, the water content of the nucleus pulposus, bright image of cerebrospinal fluid, and vertebral marrow edema (Chin, 2002). Sagittal T2-weighted images are generally best for examination of the posterior margin of the disk in relation to the neural elements (Wilmink, 1999).

As early as adolescence and routinely after age 30, an intranuclear cleft normally becomes visible on MRI. This cleft is represented by a uniformly thin band located centrally with the nucleus on T2-weighted FSE images (Morgan, 1999; Chin, 2002).

Patients with a history and physical findings consistent with disk pathology may warrant MRI for imaging of the disk and neural tissues. Presumed disk pathology may be represented by changes in signal intensity as well as in the structural relationships.

Only after considerable use of MRI has any collective agreement of terminology describing the disk evolved. A disk is considered normal if there is no extension beyond its interspace. A symmetric, diffuse extension beyond the interspace in a circumferential pattern is considered to be a disk bulge (Figure 4–24). A protrusion is characterized by a focal, asymmetric extension from the interspace; displacement of nuclear material is present, but the outer annulus fibrosus remains intact. With an extrusion, there is focal extension through all layers of the annulus fibrosus of disk material. If separation of the disk material from the parent disk occurs, a sequestration is said to be present (Fardon and Millette, 2001).

Deformity of the disk contour is most easily seen on T2-weighted images as the dark annulus fibrosus is seen in contrast to the bright cerebrospinal fluid in the thecal sac (Figure 4–25). T1-weighted images may display intermediate signal intensity, blending with the thecal sac (Maus, 2002). Sequestered fragments, if present, may be visualized more easily with gadolinium contrast administration as a peripheral ring of enhancement that typically occurs as a result of the inflammatory response elicited by the escaped nuclear material (Masaryk et al., 1988; Kazuo et al., 1993).

Intraosseous herniations of nuclear material are known as Schmorl's nodes, with most being incidental findings (Figure 4–26). They appear as extensions of disk material into

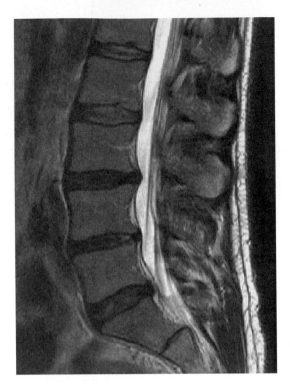

Figure 4–24 A sagittal section of a T2-weighted MRI demonstrating a bulge of multiple lumbar disks, but without clear herniation or nerve root compression. Also note the decreased signal intensity of the lower three lumbar disks compared to the upper two, consistent with degenerative change.

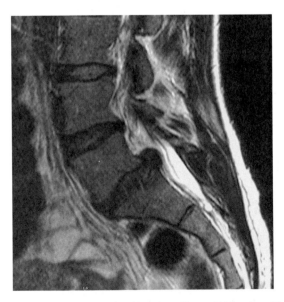

Figure 4–25 A sagittal section of a T2-weighted MRI in a 40-year-old female with a disk herniation at L5–S1 with contact and displacement of the L5 and S1 nerve roots. Also note the presence of decreased signal intensity of the disks of L4–5 and L5–S1 consistent with degenerative disease in comparison to L3–4.

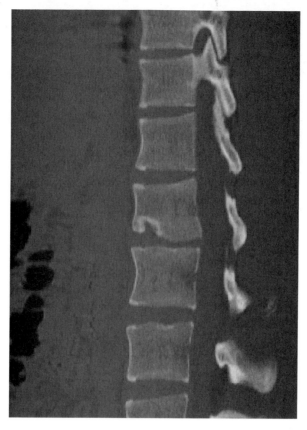

Figure 4–26 In this sagittal reconstruction CT image, the T12 vertebral body is deformed inferiorly as a result of intravertebral herniation of the disk, which is more commonly known as a Schmorl's node. MRI also effectively demonstrates these lesions.

the vertebral body, typically surrounded by a rim of low signal intensity on T1-weighted images due to reactive sclerosis and may also display marrow edema if large (Morgan and Saifuddin, 1998). T2-weighted images also demonstrate the Schmorl's nodes typical of Scheuermann's disease (Arana et al., 2002; Swischuk et al., 1998). The disorder is typified by multiple small extrusions of nuclear material through the end plates into the vertebral bodies. While only approximately 50 percent of such positive findings are painful, a predisposition to disk degeneration in later life has been documented (Arana et al., 2002; Kalifa et al., 2002).

Multiple studies (Boden et al., 1990; Jensen et al., 1994; Stadnik et al., 1998; Weishaupt et al., 1998) have documented apparent disk anomalies to occur with remarkable frequency in those individuals without any history of low back pain. Extension of the disk beyond the interspace is, therefore, not clearly pathologic and perhaps an incidental finding. Limited evidence (Boos et al., 1995; Jarvik et al., 2001) has suggested that only direct evidence of neural compression and moderate to severe stenosis occur more frequently in symptomatic individuals.

Recent limited evidence has suggested value in MRI being completed dynamically rather than in the typical supine position with hips and knees partially flexed. With axial loading, disk herniation size has been reported to be significantly increased in 21 to 50 percent of subjects (Willen and Danielson, 2001; Choy, 1997).

Similarly, positioning of the lumbar spine in either upright flexion or extension has also been suggested to have a sensitizing effect and perhaps emulating the biomechanics of the functional difficulties in patients. In a study of patients with chronic low back pain failing to respond to conservative care, annular contact with nerve root occurred in 22.4 percent of subjects while supine, but increased to 40.8 percent of subjects when imaged with seated flexion and 29.6 percent with seated extension (Weishaupt et al., 2000).

The patient with persistent difficulty following diskectomy presents a dilemma for the managing physician. MRI with gadolinium contrast is the preferred imaging modality in patients warranting further diagnostic procedures after diskectomy. Often, the diagnostic challenge is to determine if the patient's continuing difficulty is due to recurrent or continued disk pathology or fibrosis.

The annular margin may be indistinct due to tissue disruption, edema, and hemorrhage. An epidural mass effect typically occurs postoperatively, appearing very similar to the preoperative herniation (Barbar and Saiffudin, 2000). The enhancement pattern is also a factor as a recurrent or residual disk herniation typically shows no enhancement or only peripheral enhancement, but fibrosis tends to show heterogeneous enhancement (Barbar and Saiffudin, 2000; Taneichi, 2001).

MRI with contrast can identify typical patterns of arachnoiditis such as the central clumping of nerve roots, the peripheral adhesion of nerve roots to the meninges ("empty sac"), or the end-stage inflammatory mass filling the thecal sac (Ross, 2000; Barbar and Saiffudin, 2002).

Radiologists must interpret such findings with caution in the immediate postoperative period of up to 6 months due to the edema and soft tissue changes inevitably resulting from the procedure (Ross, 2000; Barbar and Saiffudin, 2002).

No other imaging modality is as informative as to the changes accompanying degeneration as MRI. The problem for the treating clinician is not in detecting degenerative changes, but in assessing the clinical relevance to the findings because of their ubiquitous presence in those of middle age and greater. Often seen before any loss of signal intensity, the earliest indications of degenerative disk disease are infolding of the anterior annular fibers and a hypointense central dot (Morgan, 1999). As the degenerative process becomes established, a generalized loss of signal intensity of the disk occurs on T2-weighted images (Chin, 2002; Morgan, 1999). Progressive degenerative disk disease is associated with further loss of signal, loss of disk height, and bulging of the annulus (Morgan, 1999). Foci of increased signal intensity may occur in degenerating disks from calcification, end plate separation, annular tears, and fluid-filled cyst spaces (Morgan, 1999; Chin, 2002). In advanced degenerative disk disease, nitrogen will collect in the intradiskal space, yielding no signal and giving rise to the vacuum disk phenomenon (Chin, 2002; Morgan, 1999) (Figure 4–27).

Degenerative disk disease evident on MRI was perhaps best described by Modic et al. (1988), which specifically details those changes seen at the end plates and the sequelae

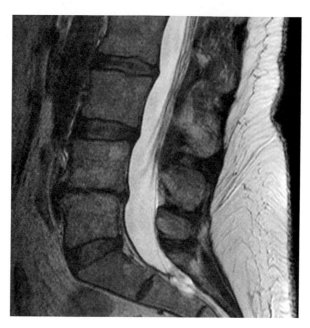

Figure 4–27 A sagittal section of a T2-weighted MRI demonstrating severe degenerative disk disease at L4–5. Note the collapse of disk space and remodeling of the adjacent bone. Bulging of the disks at neighboring levels is also present.

in the vertebral bodies. These are often referenced in imaging reports and in the literature, and the classification scheme has been found to be reliable (Jones et al., 2005). The following is a brief description (Modic et al., 1988; El-Khoury and Melhem, 2003):

Type I: Decreased signal intensity on T1-weighted and increased signal on T2-weighted images. These are generally considered to be consistent with disruption and fissuring of the end plates along with fibrovascular intrusion into the marrow. Contrast enhancement tends to occur with type I changes.

Type II: Signal intensity is increased on T1-weighted images with isointense to slightly increased signal occuring on T2-weighted images. This imaging is thought to represent fatty replacement of the vertebral body marrow adjacent to the disks.

Type III: Both T1- and T2-weighted images demonstrate decreased signal intensity, which tends to correspond to the bony sclerosis observed on radiography.

CT is superior to MRI in demonstrating bone abnormality associated with spinal trauma, but MRI exceeds all other imaging options in providing information relative to neurologic status. MRI can detect traumatic injury by obvious distortion of normal spatial relationships (Jenkins, 2001b). Excellent imaging of hemorrhage, edema, and direct visualization of the spinal cord are permitted on MRI. Thus, the role of MRI is often to identify abnormalities that underlie bony pathology (Jenkins, 2001b).

Contusion of the spinal cord is best seen on T2-weighted images with increased intramedullary signal intensity and can occur with or without fractures or dislocations. Contusions may or may not be hemorrhagic, although those with hemorrhage are typically associated with a worse prognosis (Jenkins, 2001a; Wilmink, 1999). Hemorrhage within the cord may cause signal loss on T2-weighted images (Wilmink, 1999) (Figures 4–28 and 4–29).

MRI also allows direct visualization of the ligamentous structures of the spine. When a ligament is disrupted, edematous, or hemorrhagic, it becomes uncharacteristically hyperintense on T2-weighted FSE images in the acute phase of injury (Jenkins, 2001a).

In severe trauma, the disjointed spinal canal can be clearly identified and the transected cord can be observed to float freely in the cerebrospinal fluid (Jenkins, 2001b).

While the initial findings of anklyosing spondylitis are typically evident in the sacroiliac joint, patterns characteristic of the disorder in the spine are revealed earlier in the disease process by MRI than with other imaging modalities. Typical features of the vertebral osteitis include the anterior corners of the vertebral bodies demonstrating decreased signal intensity on T1-weighted and increased signal intensity on T2-weighted images. If contrast is added, the anterior corners will be enhanced on T1-weighted images, implying active inflammation and hypervascularity. The presence of Romanus lesions ("shiny corner sign"), usually from T10 to L2, is a hallmark of the disease (Vinson and Major, 2003; Levine et al., 2004). The signal within the disk space is usually not enhanced. Andersson lesions, involving the end plates and disks, are also often revealed. On T2-weighted

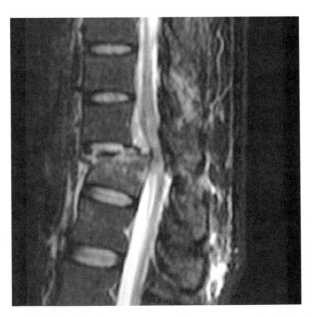

Figure 4–28 A sagittal section of a T2-weighted MRI of T12 fracture with compression of the conus medullaris. Note the obliteration of cerebrospinal fluid (CSF) signal surrounding the neural elements and patchy edema within the conus medullaris.

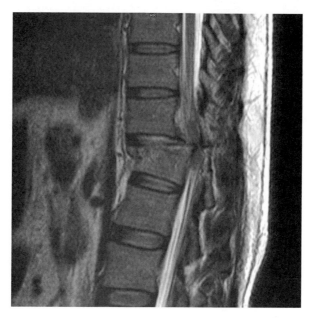

Figure 4–29 A sagittal section of a T2-weighted MRI of T12 fracture suggesting direct mechanical compression of the neural elements.

FSE images, increased signal intensity in the disk space and the surrounding bodies is displayed along with invasion of the disk material through the end plates. Signal intensity of the residual vertebral bodies and disk spaces is usually decreased on T1-weighted images and increased on T2-weighted images. Short tau inversion recovery (STIR) sequences have also been reported as being particularly effective in revealing Romanus and Andersson lesions (Hermann et al., 2005) (Figures 4–30 and 4–31).

Pseudoarthrosis usually extends to the posterior elements, and calcification of the posterior longitudinal ligament is suggested by a linear band posterior to the vertebral bodies (Vinson and Major, 2003; Levine et al., 2004).

Primary tumors of the spine occur with much less frequency than tumors from metastases, multiple myeloma, or lymphoma. MRI is the most sensitive imaging modality for the detection of most neoplastic disease (Flemming, 2000; Chin, 2002). In particular, tumors with bone marrow involvement, the soft tissues of the spine, and involving the spinal cord are best visualized by MRI. The location and signal characteristics usually allow for differential diagnosis. Primary tumors are more common in the lumbar and thoracic regions than in the cervical spine (Flemming, 2000) (Figure 4–32). T1-weighted sequences allow viewing of vertebral metastases in marrow because of the contrast in normal and abnormal tissues (Figures 4–33 and 4–34). Physicians viewing images in the elderly, however, may have difficulty differentiating pathologic and osteoporotic fractures in such disease processes (Uetani et al., 2004). Homogeneous and diffuse abnormal signal intensity along with posterior convexity and involvement of pedicles are consistent with a malignant compression fracture. A benign vertebral collapse is typically

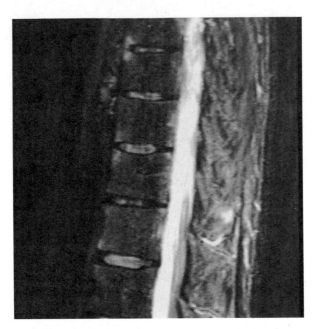

Figure 4–30 A STIR sequence sagittal slice MRI of the thoracic spine shows increased signal intensity at the anterior vertebral body edges known as Romanus lesions. *Image courtesy of Kay-Geert, A. Hermann, M. D., & RSNA Publications. Hermann, K. A, Althoff, C. E, Schneider, U, et al. (2005). Spinal changes in patients with spondyloarthritis: comparison of MR imaging and radiographic appearances. Radiographics, 25, 559–570, with permission.*

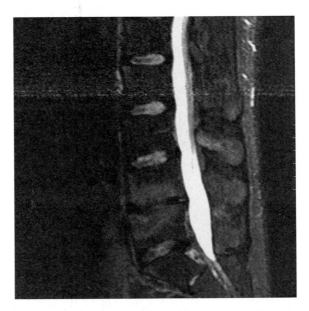

Figure 4–31 An Andersson lesion with increased signal intensity of the bone immediately surrounding the disk is demonstrated on this STIR sequence sagittal slice MRI of the lumbar spine. *Image courtesy of Kay-Geert, A. Hermann, M. D., & RSNA Publications. Hermann, K. A, Althoff, C. E, Schneider, U, et al. (2005). Spinal changes in patients with spondyloarthritis: comparison of MR imaging and radiographic appearances. Radiographics, 25, 559–570, with permission.*

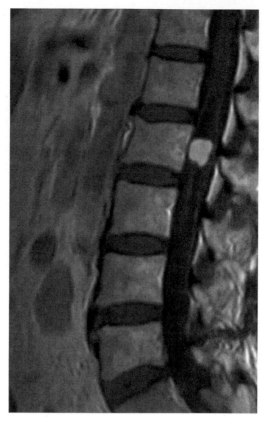

Figure 4–32 The well-defined focus of increased signal intensity in this sagittal slice contrast enhanced T1-weighted MR image is consistent with the presence of an ependymona.

demonstrated by a band-like area of low signal intensity adjacent to the depressed end plate or the signal intensity will be unchanged (Uetani et al., 2004). The addition of contrast many not help with vertebral tumors, but may assist in the visualization of epidural, intradural, and intramedullary processes (Chin, 2002).

Although infection of the spine is rare, MRI exceeds other imaging modalities in sensitivity of detection. The earliest sign in intervertebral diskitis, albeit nonspecific, is bone marrow edema. The earliest specific sign is end plate destruction as indicated by loss of definition. With progression, increased intradiskal signal intensity on T2-weighted FSE images along with disk and marrow edema are common findings (Barbar and Saiffidin, 2002; Morgan, 1999; Chin, 2002). Similarly with progression, the intranuclear cleft is no longer evident and loss of disk height becomes evident. If longstanding, the disk space can be obliterated (Chin, 2002). Suspected infection is an indication for administration of contrast for improved visualization of the epidural or paraspinal abscess usually associated with diskitis (Ross, 2000; Barbar and Saiffidin, 2002; Morgan, 1999). Infection may originate from surgery or diskography, but also from other disease processes. The most common

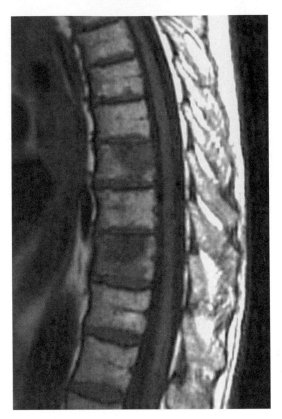

Figure 4–33 This T1-weighted sagittal section MRI reveals signal intensity changes consistent with metastases to the thoracic spine from primary lung carcinoma.

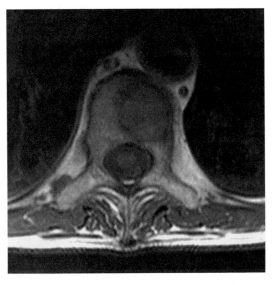

Figure 4–34 An axial T1-weighted image gives further detail of the involvement of the vertebral body from the metastatic carcinoma.

noninoculated infection is tuberculosis, typically arising from pulmonary origin. The involved vertebral bodies will usually demonstrate decreased signal intensity on T1-weighted and increased signal intensity on T2-weighted images (Lolge, 2003) (Figure 4–35). Tuberculous spondylitis usually originates in the anterior subchondral bone with the presence of extensive subligamentous spread of activity (Maus, 2002), but confirmation requires histopathologic analysis (Lolge, 2003). The destruction brought by infectious processes usually results in chronic signal changes even after effective treatment (Chin, 2002).

The use of MRI in the assessment of scoliosis has increased, but the optimal role remains yet to be defined (Redla et al., 2001). MRI offers the advantages of demonstrating concurrent intraspinal abnormalities and allows detailed imaging without ionizing radiation (Cassar-Pullicino, 2002).

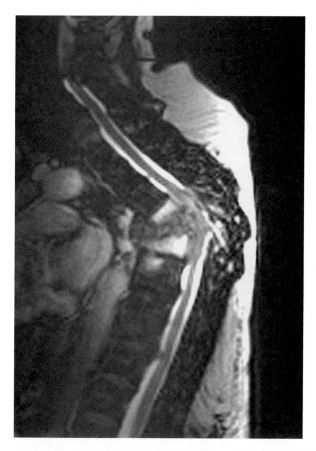

Figure 4–35 A sagittal section of T2-weighted MRI in a 54-year-old female with inflammatory diskitis. Note the abnormal signal of the neighboring vertebral bodies and gross angulation of the spine secondary to collapse of the centrally involved vertebral bodies.

DISKOGRAPHY

Diskography is conducted specifically to determine the intervertebral disk presumed to be the source of the patient's primary complaints of pain (Kapoor et al., 2003; Carino and Morrison, 2002). The prognostic value of such assertions remain incompletely studied. Thus, diskography lacks a criterion standard and has a questionable reputation based on past clinical decision making from its results (Carino and Morrison, 2002). The basic tenet of the diagnostic process is that injection into the disk and subsequent increased intradiskal pressure will elicit the patient's concordant pain (Carino and Morrison, 2002; Renfrew, 2003). The process is technically challenging for the physician and has a significant element of subjectivity given the patient's response in determining the result of the examination (Kapoor et al., 2003; Carino and Morrison, 2002). Thus, false-positive results are a concern and have been reported at rates varying from 0 to 26 percent, with particularly high rates in those with somatization disorders (Holt et al., 1968; Walsh et al., 1990; Carragee et al., 2000). To improve specificity, an attempt is often made to provide a control segment for comparison above or below the suspect disk by completing the same procedure on a presumably uninvolved disk (Kapoor et al., 2003; Carino and Morrison, 2002; Renfrew, 2003). A pressure-controlled technique has been refined in an attempt to reduce false-positive results, and early evidence suggests this may be of value (O'Neill and Kurgansky, 2004). Further information is obtained by completion of a CT scan to observe the contrast distribution within the disk to provide a probable correlation to disruption of the annulus (Kapoor et al., 2003; Renfrew, 2003) (Figures 4–36 and 4–37).

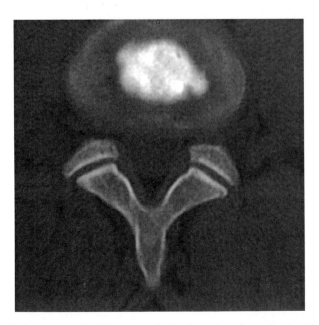

Figure 4–36 In this image of a CT diskogram in the lumbar spine, the contrast material is contained within the central portion of the disk, suggesting intact structure.

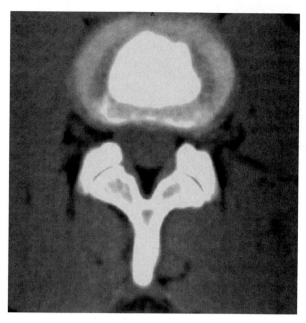

Figure 4–37 In this CT diskogram image, the contrast material is extravasated posteriorly between the lamellae of the annulus, consistent with separation of those layers.

Much of the current controversy with diskography is in the investigation of possible internal disk disruption as a source of pain, which may or may not be readily revealed on MRI (Kapoor et al., 2003). Internal disk disruption is generally considered to consist of derangement of the nucleus and annular lamellae of the disk, particularly with radial fissuring, while the outer structure is not significantly altered. As such, neurologic status is not altered as often occurs with disk herniation. A recent literature review, however, reveals that firm diagnostic criteria have yet to be agreed upon (Lee et al., 2003). Evidence is conflicting as to the degree of correspondence between positive findings of internal disk disruption at diskography and a hyperintense zone on MRI T2-weighted images (Lam et al., 2000; Brightbill et al., 1994; Aprill et al., 1992). The nature of internal disk disruption is, however, incompletely understood, and its relationship to painful lumbar syndromes has yet to be established (Lee et al., 2003).

A significant consideration with diskography with injection of the disk, as opposed to MRI, is the invasiveness of the procedure. Risk of diskitis subsequent to diskography has been estimated at 1 to 4 percent (Carino and Morrison, 2002).

 IMAGING RELATING TO OSTEOPOROSIS

With osteoporosis potentially affecting multiple decisions made by the rehabilitation professional, an understanding of bone densiometry is essential. Dual energy x-ray absorptiometry (DEXA) consists of two x-ray energies absorbed differentially as a means of assessing and monitoring bone density. DEXA is generally considered the gold standard for bone densiometry owing to the extent to which it has been validated against fracture outcomes (Nelson et al., 2002). Applied particularly as a portion of a monitoring or treatment program, DEXA is the best predictor of fracture risk associated with osteoporosis (Ahrar et al., 2002; Westmacott, 1995). DEXA is a much more sensitive method of examining bone density than radiography, while allowing for less radiation exposure and rapid image acquisition (Guermazi et al., 2002). Vertebral fractures due to osteoporosis are underdiagnosed by radiography with false-negative rates of 27 to 45 percent (Guermazi et al., 2002). Additionally, the precision of DEXA allows for easier sequential examinations in follow-up during prevention and treatment approaches (Lentle and Prior, 2003). Measures are site specific to some degree, requiring the spine and proximal femur be assessed individually for their clinical relevance (Ahrar et al., 2002). Other rapid methods of assessment of bone mineral density, including ultrasound, are available, but DEXA is the most widely used method in North America (Ahrar et al., 2002; Westmacott, 1995) (Figure 4–38).

The diagnosis of osteoporosis is largely dependent upon the DEXA quantification of bone density in criteria put forth by the World Health Organization (WHO, 1994). The T-score is in reference to the number of standard deviations from the mean of healthy, young adults (Table 4–3).

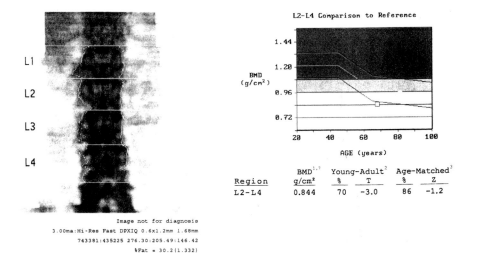

Figure 4–38 An example of a dual energy x-ray absorptiometry (DEXA) report. Note the T-score value of 3.0, which is categorized as osteoporosis according to the World Health Organization definition.

TABLE 4–3	DEXA Quantification of Bone Density in Criteria put Forth by the World Health Organization
Classification	**Bone Mineral Density (t-score)**
Normal	+2.5 to −1.0
Osteopenia or low bone mineral density	−1.0 to −2.5
Osteoporosis	≤ − 2.5
Severe osteoporosis	≤ − 2.5 plus fragility fracture

Derived as data from WHO, 1994. 21

Rehabilitation professionals may also encounter patients having undergone procedures to address vertebral compression resulting from osteoporosis. Vertebroplasty and kyphoplasty are attempts to stabilize the structure of the vertebral body (Figures 4–39 to 4–42). Kyphoplasty also offers the attempt toward restoration of vertebral body height, thereby potentially affecting overall posture and alignment. Images before and after the procedures are typical.

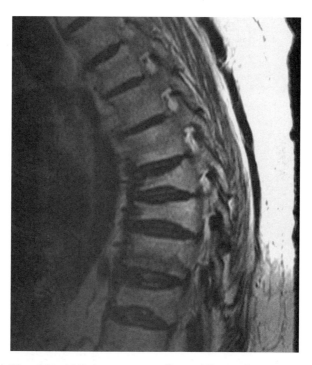

Figure 4–39 This T1-weighted MR demonstrates collapse of the vertebrae as associated with osteoporotic fractures.

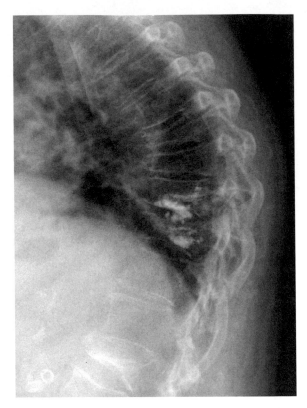

Figure 4–40 A lateral view radiograph of the same patient following injection into the involved vertebral bodies of polymethyl methacrylate. Note the radiolucency of the surrounding vertebrae due to demineralization.

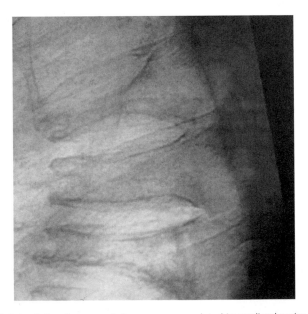

Figure 4–41 This lateral view fluoroscopic image was completed immediately prior to kyphoplasty.

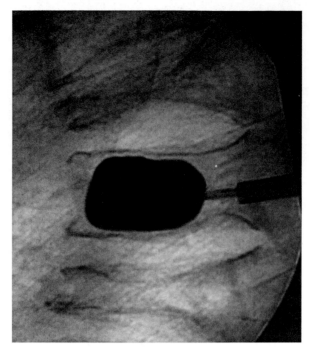

Figure 4–42 In this image captured during the kyphoplasty procedure, a balloon is enlarged within the vertebral body to reverse the wedging. The vertebral body is then stabilized by injection of polymethyl methacrylate within the cavity formed by the balloon. Note the reduction in wedging with expansion of the balloon.

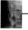 ## ULTRASOUND

An aspect to imaging in which those in rehabilitation are directly involved is the use of ultrasound to examine the function of the lumbopelvic stabilizing musculature. Of particular interest are the lumbar multifidus and transversus abdominis with efforts to assist in feedback for improved activation of this target musculature for therapeutic exercise. Difficulties with recruitment of the lumbar multifidus and transversus abdominis have been documented in patients with low back pain compared to asymptomatic individuals (Hodges et al., 1996; Hides et al., 1994). Specific exercise programs have subsequently been developed based on selective activation of this musculature (O'Sullivan et al., 1997; Richardson et al., 2004). The basis of this effort is to assist the patient with low back pain to gain better motor control of the supporting musculature to address the immediate and longer term self-management needs.

In this application, ultrasound imaging is used to demonstrate selective thickening of the targeted transversus abdominis and lumbar multifidus and, thus, the desired pattern

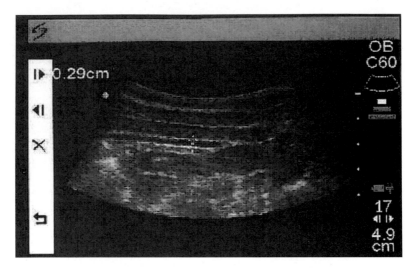

Figure 4–43 This ultrasound image demonstrates the abdominal musculature at rest.

of muscle recruitment thought to be important in the rehabilitation process (Henry and Westervelt, 2005; Teyhen et al., 2005). The results of ultrasound imaging have been found consistent with MRI findings of increased muscle thickness during attempts at selective activation (Hides et al., 2006). The preponderance of evidence to date has been favorable as to the value of this imaging methodology. Trials with patients experiencing low back pain

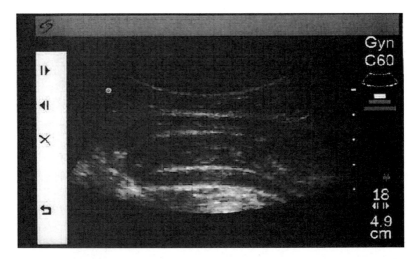

Figure 4–44 With an attempt to activate the transversus abdominis musculature, a compensatory increase in the internal oblique musculature is apparent, suggesting a suboptimal activation pattern.

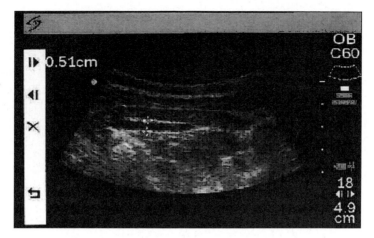

Figure 4–45 This image displays the increase in thickness of the transversus abdominis musculature. Note the absence of a compensatory increase in thickness of the internal oblique musculature.

and controls have demonstrated enhanced learning and improved performance retention of activation of the target stabilizing musculature (Henry and Westervelt, 2005; Kiesel et al., 2006; Worth et al., 2007; Van et al., 2006). A similar study by Teyhen et al. (2005), however, failed to establish similarly improved learning patterns by patients (Figures 4–43 to 4–47). This developing area of interest will unquestionably be investigated more thoroughly in the near future with the value of rehabilitative ultrasound imaging to be clarified.

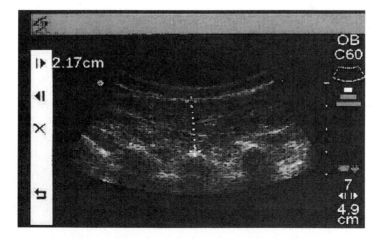

Figure 4–46 A parasagittal view of the lumbar multifidus musculature at rest.

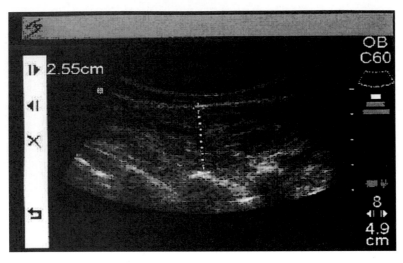

Figure 4–47 This parasagittal view of the lumbar multifidi is during voluntary activation, demonstrating an increase in size from 2.17 cm at rest to 2.55 cm activation.

 ## CLINICAL RELEVANCE TO PHYSICAL THERAPY

Rehabilitation Implications 1

For clinicians routinely providing care for patients presenting with complaints of low back pain, incorporating diagnostic imaging results into the clinical decision making process can be a challenge.

For the adult patient presenting with low back pain without traumatic onset, radiography is declining in use. Though sometimes reassuring to the patient, the results yielded by conventional radiography images are typically of little value in clinical decision making. As most mechanical low back pain, particularly in the acute phase, is associated with a soft tissue origin, imaging sensitivities and specificities for detection of the pain origin with plain radiography are usually noncontributory to the clinician's overall understanding of the patient. Thus, physicians are justifiably utilizing this imaging modality less under such circumstances. Patients unfamiliar with imaging modality strengths and weaknesses frequently misinterpret this omission. Similarly, while MRI may or may not offer identification of pathology, the results often do not change the course of care initially. These considerations are particularly relevant to physical therapists as decisions are usually based on detailed clinical examination findings and observations rather than imaging results.

Exceptions in this generalization to the value of radiography for the examination of patients with acute low back pain in initial decision making exist. Patients with other medical conditions or histories elevating the risk for significant findings may require imaging initially to determine appropriateness for physical therapy participation. Adolescents with low back pain, often due to spondylolysis or spondylolisthesis, may require radiographic imaging before appropriateness for physical therapy can be determined.

Full knowledge of the patient's medical and current contributing histories as well as communication with the physician providing care are imperative to appropriate decision making by the physical therapist.

Rehabilitation Implications 2

Radiography is often the first line of diagnostic imaging chosen when investigation for a compression fracture is undertaken. While such injuries are usually identifiable on plain film radiography, further investigation may be warranted if interpretations are negative yet clinical suspicion continues. Postmenopausal females or females with other predisposing medical conditions warrant particular caution with decision making. As any mechanical treatment option must be explored with caution in such patients, physical therapists must have reasonable assurance that no fracture is present before addressing patients with interscapular, thoracic, or thoracolumbar area pain. This is especially pertinent if risk factors such as age, gender, concurrent medical conditions, medication usage, and prior history align to accumulate an elevated risk for fracture.

 ## ADDITIONAL READING

Bogduk, N., & Modic, M. T. (1996). Lumbar discography. *Spine, 21,* 402–404.

McKinnis, L. N. (1997*). Fundamentals of orthopedic radiology.* Philadelphia; Davis.

Weishaupt, D., Zanetti, M., Hodler, J., et al. (2001). Painful lumbar disk derangement: relevance of endplate abnormalities at MR imaging. *Radiology, 218,* 420–427.

 ## REFERENCES

Adam, C., Izatt, M., Harvey, J., & Askin G. (2005). Variability in Cobb angle measurements using reformatted computerized tomography scans. *Spine, 30,* 1664–1669.

Ahrar, K., Schomer, D., & Wallace, M. J. (2002). Kyphoplasty for the treatment of vertebral compression fractures. *Seminars in Interventional Radiology, 10,* 235–244.

Alfieri, K. M., & Hesselink, J. R. (1997). MR imaging of spinal stenosis. *Applied Radiology, Aug,* 18–27.

Aprill, C., & Bogduk, N. (1992). High-intensity zone: a diagnostic sign of painful lumbar disc on magnetic resonance imaging. *British Journal of Radiology, 65,* 361–369.

Arana, E., Marti-Bonmati, L., Dosda, R., & Molla, E. (2002). Concomitant lower thoracic disc disease in lumbar spine MR imaging studies. *European Radiology, 12,* 2794–2798.

Arslantas, A., Atasoy, M. A., Guner, A.I., et al. (2002). Three dimensional computed tomography in spinal pathologies. *Radiography, 8,* 173–179.

Barbar, S., & Saifuddin, A. (2002). MRI of the post-discectomy spine. *Clinical Radiology, 57,* 969–981.

Bensch, F. V., Kiuru, M. J., Koivikko, M. P., & Koskinen S.K. (2004). Spine fractures in falling accidents: analysis of multidetector CT findings. *European Radiology, 14,* 618–624.

Boden, S. D., Davis, D. O, Dina, T. S., et al. (1990). Abnormal magnetic-resonance scans of the lumbar spine in asymptomatic subjects. *Journal of Bone and Joint Surgery (American), 72,* 403–408.

Bolender, N. F., Schonstrom, N. S., & Spengler, D. M. & (1985). Lumbar vertebral canal morphometry for computerized tomography in spinal stenosis. *Journal of Bone and Joint Surgery (American), 67,* 240–246.

Boos, N., Rieder, R., Schade, V., et al. (1995). Volvo award in the clinical sciences: the diagnostic accuracy of magnetic resonance imaging, work perception, and psychosocial factors in identifying symptomatic disc herniation. *Spine, 20,* 2613–2625.

Brightbill, T. C., Pile, N., Eichelberger, R. P., & Whitman, M., Jr. (1994). Normal magnetic resonance imaging and abnormal discography in lumbar disc disruption. *Spine, 19,* 1075–1077.

Carino, J. A., & Morrison, W. B. (2002). Discography: current concepts and techniques. *Applied Radiology, Aug,* 32–40.

Carragee, E., Tanner, C., Khurana, S., et al. (2000). The rates of false positive findings on lumbar discography in selected patients without low back symptoms. *Spine, 25,* 1373–1381.

Cassar-Pullicino, V. N., Eisenstein, S. M. (2002). Imaging in scoliosis: what, why and how. *Clinical Radiology, 57,* 543–562.

Chin, C.T. (2002). Spine imaging. *Seminars in Neurology, 22,* 205–220.

Choy, D. S. (1997). Magnetic resonance imaging of the lumbosacral spine under compression. *Journal of Clinical Laser Medicine & Surgery, 15,* 71–73.

Curylo, L. J., Edwards C., & DeWald RW. (2002). Radiographic markers in spondyloptosis: implications for spondylolisthesis progression. *Spine, 27,* 2021–2025.

Collins, J. Chest wall trauma. *Journal of Thoracic Imaging, 15,* 112–119.

Cortet, B., Roches, E., Logier, R., et al. (2002). Evaluation of spinal curvatures after a recent osteoporotic vertebral fracture. *Joint, Bone, Spine, 69,* 201–208.

Christensen, F. (2004). Lumbar spinal fusion. Outcome in relation to surgical methods, choice of implant and postoperative rehabilitation. *Acta Orthopaedica Scandinavica Supplement, 75,* 2–43.

Dai, L., Yao, W., Cui, Y, & Zhou, Q. (2004). Thoracolumbar fractures in patients with multiple injuries: diagnosis and treatment-a review of 147 cases. *Journal of Trauma, 56,* 348–355.

Denis, F. (1983). The three column spine and its significance in the classification of acute thoracolumbar spinal injuries. *Spine, 8,* 817–831.

Dupuis, P., Yong-Hing, K., Cassidy, J., & Kirkaldy-Willis, W. (1985). Radiologic diagnosis of degenerative lumbar spine instability. *Spine, 10,* 262–276.

El-Khoury, GY., Bennett, DL., & Stanley, MD. (2003). Essentials of musculoskeletal imaging. Philadelphia, Churchill Livingstone.

Erkula, G., & Sponseller, P. D., & Kiter, A. E. (2003). Rib deformity in scoliois. *European Spine Journal, 12,* 281–287.

Fardon, D. F., & Millette, P. C. (2002). Nomenclature and classification of lumbar disc pathology. *Spine, 26,* E93–113.

Flemming, D. J., Murphy, M. D., Carmichael, B. B., & Bernard, S. A. (2000). Primary tumors of the spine. *Seminars in Musculoskeletal Radiology, 4,* 299–320.

Fujiwara, A., Tamai, K., An, H., et al. (2000). The relationship between disc degeneration, facet joint osteoarthritis, and stability of the degenerative lumbar spine. *Journal of Spinal Disorders, 13,* 444–450.

Fukuda, K., & Kawakami, G. (2001). Proper use of MR imaging for evaluation of low back pain. *Seminars in Musculoskeletal Radiology, 5,* 133–136.

Gillan, MG., Gilbert, FJ., Andrew, JE., Grant, AM., Wardlaw, D., Valentine, NW., Gregori, AC., & Scottish Back Trial Group. (2001). Influence of imaging on clinical decision making in the treatment of lower back pain. *Radiology, 220,* 393–99.

Gran, J., & Skomsvoll, J. (1997). The outcome of ankylosing spondylitis: a study of 100 patients. *British Journal of Rheumatology, 36,* 766–771.

Greenspan, A. (2000). *Orthopedic radiology.* 3rd ed. Philadelphia: Lippincott Williams & Wilkins.

Grigoryan, M., Roemer, F., Mohr, A., & Genant, H. (2004). Imaging in spondyloarthropathies. *Current Rheumatology Reports, 6,* 102–109.

Guermazi, A., Mohn, A., Grigorian, M., et al. (2002). Identification of vertebral fractures in osteoporosis. *Seminars in Musculoskeletal Radiology, 6,* 241–252.

Hanley, S. D., Gun, M. T., Osti, O., & Shanahan, E. M. (1999). Radiology of intervertebral cages in spinal surgery. *Clinical Radiology, 54,* 201–206.

Henry, S. M., & Westervelt, K. C. (2005). The use of real time ultrasound feedback in teaching abdominal hollowing exercises to healthy subjects. *Journal of Orthopaedic and Sports Physical Therapy, 35,* 338–345.

Hermann, K.-G., Althoff, C. E., Schneider, U., et al. (2005). Spinal changes in patients with spondyloarthritis: comparison of MR imaging and radiographic appearances. *Radiographics, 25,* 559–570.

Herzog, C., Ahle, H., Mack, M. G., et al. (2004). Traumatic injuries to the pelvis and thoracic and lumbar spine: does thin-slice multidetector-row CT increase diagnostic accuracy? *European Radiology, 14,* 1751–1760.

Hides, J., Wilson, S., Stanton, W., et al. (2006). An MRI investigation into the function of the transversus abdominis muscle during "drawing-in" of the abdominal wall. *Spine, 31,* E175–178.

Hides, J. A., Stokes, M. J., Saide, M., et al. (1994). Evidence of lumbar multifidus muscle wasting ipsilateral to symptoms in patients with acute/subacute low back pain. *Spine, 19,* 165–172.

Hirai, T., Korogi, Y., Takahashi, M., & Shimomura, O. (2001). Ossification of the posterior longitudinal ligament and ligamentum flavum: imaging features. *Seminars in Musculoskeletal Radiology, 5,* 83–88.

Hodges, P. W., & Richardson, C. A. (1996). Inefficient muscular stabilization of the lumbar spine associated with low back pain. A motor control evaluation of transversus abdominis. *Spine, 21,* 2640–2650.

Holmes, J. F., Miller, P. Q, Panacek, E. A., et al. (2001). Epidemiology of thoracolumbar spine injury in blunt trauma. *Academy of Emergency Medicine, 8,* 866–872.

Holt, EP. (1968). The question of lumbar discography. *Journal of Bone and Joint Surgery (American), 50,* 720–726.

Howland, W. J., Curry, J. L., & Buffington, C. P. (1965). Fulcrum fractures of the lumbar spine. Transverse fractures induced by an improperly placed seatbelt. *JAMA, 193,* 240–241.

Iguchi, T., Kanemura, A., Kasahara K., et al. (2004). Lumbar instability and clinical symptoms: which is the more critical for symptoms: sagittal translation or segment angulation. *Journal of Spinal Disorders & Techniques, 17,* 284–290.

Imhof, H., & Fuchsjäger, M. (2002). Traumatic injuries: imaging spinal injuries. *European Radiology, 12,* 1262–1272.

Jarvik, J. J., Hollingwort, H., Heagerty, P., et al. (2001). The longitudinal assessment of imaging and disability of the back. *Spine, 26,* 1158–1166.

Jensen, M. C., Brant-Zawadzki, M. N., Obuchowski, N., et al. (1994). Magnetic resonance imaging of the lumbar spine in people without back pain. *New England Journal of Medicine, 331,* 69–73.

Jinkins, J. R. (2001a). MR of spinal trauma: part 1. *Applied Radiology, April,* 36–44.

Jinkins, J. R. (2001b). MR of spinal trauma: part 2. *Applied Radiology, June,* 25–29.

Jones, A., Clark, A., Freeman, B., et al. (2005). The Modic classification: inter- and intraobserver error in clinical practice. *Spine, 30,* 1867–1869.

Khan, M. (2002). Thoughts concerning the early diagnosis of ankylosing spondylitis and related diseases. *Clinical and Experimental Rheumatology, 20,* S6–10.

Kalifa, G., Cohen P. A., & Hamidou, A. (2002). The intervertebral disk: a landmark for spinal diseases in children. *European Radiology, 12,* 660–665.

Kapoor, V., Rothfus, W. E., & Grahovac, S. Z. (2003). Simplified approach to discography: two triangles and a box. *Applied Radiology, January* (supplement), 23–27.

Kauppila, L., Eustace, S., Kiel, D., et al. (1998). Degenerative displacement of lumbar vertebrae. A 25 year follow-up study in Framingham. *Spine, 23,* 1868–1873.

Kazuo, Y, Kazuo, H., & Akihiko, K. (1993). Gadolinium-DTPA enhanced magnetic resonance imaging of a sequestered lumbar intervertebral disc and its correlation with pathologic findings. *Spine, 19,* 479–482.

Khoo, LA., Heron, C., Patel, U., Given-Wilson, R., Grundy, A., Know, KT., & Dundas, D. (2003). The diagnostic contribution of the frontal lumbar spine radiograph in community referred low back pain—a prospective study of 1030 patients. *Clinical Radiol, 58,* 606–609

Kiesel, K., Underwood, F., Mattacola, C., & Nitz, A. (2006). *A comparison of select trunk muscle thickness change between subjects with acute low back pain classified in the treatment-based classification system and asymptomatic controls.* Lexington: University of Kentucky.

Kifune, M., Panjabi, M. M., Liu, W., et al. (1997). Functional morphology of the spinal canal after endplate, wedge, and burst fractures. *Journal of Spinal Disorders, 10,* 457–466.

Kuhlman, J. E., Pozniak, M. A., Collins, J., & Knisely, B. L. (1998). Radiographic and CT findings of blunt chest trauma: aortic injuries and looking beyond them. *Radiographics, 18,* 1085–1106.

Lam, K. S., Carlin, D., & Mulholland, R. C. (2000). Lumbar disc high intensity zone: the value and significance of provocative discography in the determination of the discogenic pain source. *European Spine Journal, 9,* 36–41.

Lee, K. S., Doh, J. W., Bae, H. G., & Yun I. G. (2003). Diagnostic criteria for the clinical syndrome of internal disc disruption: are they reliable? *British Journal of Neurosurgery, 17,* 19–23.

Levine, D. S., Forbat, S. M., & Saifuddin, A. (2004). MRI of the axial skeleton manifestations of ankylosing spondylitis. *Clinical Radiology, 59,* 400–413.

Lentle, B. C., & Prior, J. C. (2003). Osteoporosis: what a clinician expects to learn from a patient's bone density examination. *Radiology, 228,* 620–628.

Lolge, S., Maheshwari, M., Shah, J., et al. (2003). Isolated solitary vertebral body tuberculosis—study of seven cases. *Clinical Radiology, 58,* 545–550.

Maigne, J., Lapeyre, E., Morvan, G., & Chatellier, G. (2003). Pain immediately upon sitting down and relieved by standing up is often associated with radiologic lumbar instability or marked anterior loss of disc space. *Spine, 28,* 1327–1334.

Masaryk, T., Ross, J., Modic, M., et al. (1998). MR imaging of sequestered lumbar intervertebral disks. *American Journal of Roentgenology, 150,* 1155–1162.

Maus, T. Imaging of the spine and nerve roots. *Physical Medicine and Rehabilitation Clinics of North America, 13,* 487–544.

McAfee, P. C., Hansen, Y. A., Fredrickson, B. E., et al. (1983). The value of computed tomography in thoracolumbar fractures. *Journal of Bone and Joint Surgery (American), 65,* 461–473.

Meyerding, HW. (1932). Spondylisthesis. *Surg Gynecol Obstet,* 54, 371–77.

Modic, M., Masaryk, T., Ross, J., & Carter, J. Imaging of degenerative disk disease. *Radiology, 168,* 177–86.

Morgan, S., & Saifuddin, A. (1999). MRI of the lumbar intervertebral disc. *Clinical Radiology, 54,* 703–723.

Nelson, H., Helfand, M., Woolf, S., & Allan, J. (2002). Screening for postmenopausal osteoporosis: a review of evidence for the U.S. Preventive Services task force. *Annals of Internal Medicine, 137,* 529–541.

O'Neill, C., & Kurgansky, M. (2004). Subgroups of positive discs on discography. *Spine, 29,* 2134–9.

O'Sullivan, P. B., Phyty, G. D., Twomey, L. T., & Allison, G. T. (1997). Evaluation of specific stabilizing exercise in the treatment of chronic low back pain with radiologic diagnosis of spondylolysis or spondylolisthesis. *Spine, 22,* 2959–2967.

Pathria, M. (2005). Imaging of spine instability. *Seminars in Musculoskeletal Radiology, 9,* 88–99.

Peterson, CK., Bolton, JE., & Wood, AR. (2000). A cross-sectional study correlating lumbar spine degeneration with disability and pain. *Spine,* 25, 218–23.

Pitanken, M. T., Manninen, H. I, Lindgren, K.A., et al. (2002). Segmental lumbar spine instability at flexion-extension radiography can be predicted by conventional radiography. *Clinical Radiology, 57,* 632–639.

Quek, S. T., & Peh, W. C. (2002). Radiology of osteoporosis. *Seminars in Musculoskeletal Radiology, 6,* 197–206.

Redla, S., Dar, T., & Saifuddin, A. Magnetic resonance imaging of scoliosis. *Clinical Radiology, 56,* 360–371.

Renfrew, D. (2003). Diskography. In El-Khoury, G. (ed.). *Essentials of musculoskeletal imaging.* Philadelphia: Churchill Livingstone.

Richardson, C., Hodges, P., & Hides, J. A. (2004). *Therapeutic exercise for lumbopelvic stabilization: a motor control approach for the treatment and prevention of low back pain.* 2nd ed. St. Louis: Churchill Livingstone.

Ross, J. (2002). Magnetic resonance imaging of the postoperative spine. *Seminars in Musculoskeletal Radiology, 4,* 281–292.

Rossi, F., & Dragoni, S. (2001). The prevalence of spondylolisthesis and spondylolysis in symptomatic elite athletes: radiographic findings. *Radiography, 7,* 37–42.

Saifuddin, A. (2000). The imaging of lumbar spinal stenosis. *Clinical Radiology, 55,* 581–594.

Saiffudin, A., & Hassan, A. (2003). Paget's disease of the spine: Unusual features and complicatons. *Clinical Radiology, 58,* 102–111.

Saifuddin, A., Blease, S., & MacSweeney, E. (2003). Loaded MRI of the lumbar spine. *Clinical Radiology, 58,* 661–671.

Sampaio-Barros, P., Bertolo, M., Kraemer, M., et al. (2001). Primary ankylosing spondylitis: patterns of disease in a Brazilian population of 147 patients. *Journal of Rheumatology, 28,* 560–565.

Savitsky, E., & Votey, S. (1997). Emergency department approach to acute thoracolumbar spine injury. *Journal of Emergency Medicine, 15,* 49–60.

Schwab, F., el-Fegoun, A., Gamez, L., et al. (2005). A lumbar classification of scoliosis in the adult patient: preliminary approach. *Spine, 30,* 1670–1673.

Shea, K., Stevens, P., Nelson, M., et al. (1998). A comparison of manual versus computer-assisted radiographic measurement: intraobserver measurement variability. *Spine, 23,* 551–555.

Sheridan, R., Peralta, R., Rhea, J., et al. (2003). Reformatted visceral protocol helical computed tomographic scanning allows conventional radiographs of the thoracic and lumbar spine to be eliminated in the evaluation of blunt trauma patients. *Journal of Trauma, 55,* 665–669.

Simmons, ED., Guy, RD., Graham-Smith, A., & Herzog, R. (2003). Radiograph assessment for patients with low back pain. *The Spine Journal,* 3, 3–5.

Stadnik, T. W., Lee, R. R., Cohen, H. L., et al. (1998). Annular tears and disk herniation; prevalence and contrast enhancement on MR images in the absence of low back pain or sciatica. *Radiology, 206,* 49–55.

Steinberg, E. L., Luger, E., Arbel, R., et al. (2003). A comparative roentgenographic analysis of the lumbar spine in male army recruits with and without lower back pain. *Clinical Radiology, 58,* 985–989.

Swischuk, L. E., John, S. D., & Allberry, S. (1998).: Disk degenerative disease in childhood: Scheuermann's disease, Schmorl's nodes, and the limbus vertebra: MRI findings in 12 patients. *Pediatric Radiology, 28,* 334–338.

Sys, J., Michielsen, J., Bracke, P., et al. (2001). Nonoperative treatment of active spondylolysis in elite athletes with normal x-ray findings: literature review and results of conservative treatment. *European Spine Journal, 10,* 498–504.

Taneichi, H. (2001). Role of MR imaging in the evaluation of low back pain: an orthopedic surgeon's view. *Seminars in Musculoskeletal Radiology, 5,* 129–132.

Taillard, WF. (1976). Etiology of spondylolisthesis. *Clinical Orthopaedics and Related Research,* 117, 30–39.

Teyhen, D. S., Miltenberger, C. E., et al. (2005). The use of ultrasound imaging of the abdominal drawing-in maneuver in subjects with low back pain. *Journal of Orthopaedic and Sports Physical Therapy, 35,* 346–355.

Torgenson, WR., & Dotler, WE. (1976). Comparative roentgenographic study of the asymptomatic and symptomatic lumbar spine. *Journal of Bone and Joint Surgery—American,* 58, 850—853.

Uetani, M., Hashmi, R., & Hayashi, K. (2004). Malignant and benign compression fractures: differentiation and diagnostic pitfalls on MRI. *Clinical Radiology, 59,* 124–131.

Van den Bosch, M. A., Hollingworth, W., Kinmouth A. L., & Dixon, A. K. (2004). Evidence against the use of lumbar spine radiography for low back pain. *Clinical Radiology, 59,* 69–76.

Vinson, E. N., & Major, N. M. (2003). MR imaging of anklyosing spondylitis. *Seminars in Musculoskeletal Radiology, 7,* 103–114.

Van, K., Hides, J., & Richardson, C. The use of real-time ultrasound imaging for biofeedback of lumbar multifidus muscle contraction in healthy subjects. *Journal of Orthopaedic and Sports Physical Therapy, 36,* 920–925.

Verbiest, H. (1977). Results of surgical treatment of idiopathic developmental stenosis of the lumbar vertebral canal. A review of twenty-seven years' experience. *Journal of Bone and Joint Surgery (British), 59,* 181–188.

Vollmer, D., & Gegg, C. (1997). Classification and acute management of thoracolumbar fractures. *Neurosurgery Clinics of North America, 8,* 499–507.

Walsh, T., Weinstein, J., Spratt, K., et al. (1990). Lumbar discography in normal subjects. *Journal of Bone and Joint Surgery (American), 72,* 72:1081–1088.

Weishaupt, D., Schmid, M., Zanetti, M., et al. (2000). Positional MR imaging of the lumbar spine: does it demonstrate nerve root compromise not visible at conventional MR imaging. *Radiology, 215,* 247–253.

Weishaupt, D., Zanetti, M., Hodler, J., et al. (1998). MR imaging of the lumbar spine: prevalence of intervertebral disc extrusion and sequestration, nerve root compression, end plate abnormalities, and osteoarthritis of the facet joint in asymptomatic volunteers. *Radiology, 209,* 661–666.

Weisz, G. M., & Lee, P. (1983). Spinal canal stenosis. Concept of spinal reserve capacity: radiologic measurements and clinical applications. *Clinical Orthopaedics and Related Research, 179,* 134–140.

Westmacott, C. F. (1995). Osteoporosis-what is it, how is it measured and what can be done about it? *Radiography, 1,* 35–47.

White, A. A., & Panjabi, M. M. (1990). *Clinical biomechanics of the spine.* 2nd ed. Philadelphia: Lippincott.

Wilmink, J, T. (1999). MR imaging of the spine: trauma and degenerative disease. *European Radiology, 9,* 1259–1266.

Willen, J., & Danielson, B. (2001). The diagnostic effect from axial loading of the lumbar spine during computed tomography and magnetic resonance imaging in patients with degenerative disorders. *Spine, 26,* 2607–2614.

Wimberly, R. L., & Lauerman, W. C. (2002). Spondylolisthesis in the athlete. *Clinical Sports Medicine, 21,* 133–145.

Wintermark, M., Mouhsine, E., Theumann, N., et al. (2003). Thoracolumbar spine fractures in patients who have sustained severe trauma: depiction with multi-detector row CT. *Radiology, 227,* 681–689.

Witt, I., Vestergaard, A., & Rosenklint, A. (1984). A comparative analysis of x-ray findings of the lumbar spine in patients with and without lumbar pain. *Spine, 9,* 298–300.

WHO (1994). *Assessment of fracture risk and its application to screening for postmenopausal osteoporosis.* WHO Technical Report Series 843. Geneva: World Health Organization.

Worth, S., Henry, S., & Bunn, J. (2007). Real-time ultrasound feedback and abdominal hollowing exercises for people with low back pain. *New Zealand Journal of Physiotherapy, 35,* 4–11.

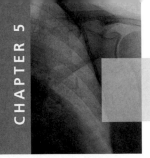

CHAPTER 5

Shoulder Complex

Imaging of the shoulder remains a challenge primarily related to the multiple layers of overlapping soft and bony tissues. Often an image reflects not only the single structure but rather that structure superimposed onto several other structures. This leads to numerous "special" projections which attempt to better isolate the desired structure. Much like imaging of the knee, clinicians increasingly have begun to use magnetic resonance imaging (MRI) as a more definitive modality again directly through its ability to provide both soft tissue and bony differentiations.

The shoulder is the most mobile joint in the body and is composed of a true complex of both bony and soft tissue articulations. A very appropriate description is that the shoulder is designed to provide mobility with stability being secondary (at best). The bony components are the humerus, scapula, and clavicle, while the soft tissue articulation is that of the scapula and thorax (scapulothoracic joint).

The clavicle serves as a crankshaft-strut assembly maintaining the ability of the arm to be positioned functionally while doing so in an efficient fashion. The clavicle is often the victim of falls onto the shoulder or direct trauma associated with vehicles, particularly bicycles.

The scapula is positioned by soft tissues to permit appropriate function of the arm through orientation of the glenoid in relation to the humeral head. This finely tuned process is described as scapulohumeral rhythm and provides the harmonious functions of the upper extremity while enabling it to be anchored to the trunk. The scapulothoracic joint provides an upward rotation and sliding movement which requires a well-orchestrated sequence of proximal muscular actions in concert with humeral rotators (actually centering/compressing the humeral head onto the glenoid) and humeral movers culminating in upper extremity functional actions. The superior projection of the scapula includes the acromion which provides the "roof" of the glenohumeral joint proper, while the inferior projection is the coracoid process serving as an anchor for muscle and ligament insertions.

The humerus provides the proximal rounded head which articulates with the rather flat glenoid fossa of the scapula (Figure 5–1). Thus the round head sitting/positioned onto a flat "saucer" provides an inherently unstable glenohumeral joint which is also dictated by the small size of the glenoid as well. The glenoid labrum is a fibrocartilagenous rim which helps increase the contact between these structures by enhancing the peripheral surface thickness much as does the meniscus of the knee. Although very dense, only special image modalities well define this wedge-shaped fibrous structure, with MRI being most typically being applied today.

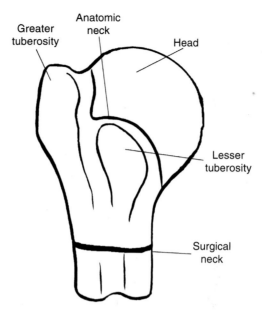

Figure 5–1 The features of the proximal humerus in contribution to the glenohumeral articulation.

The space between the humeral head and the acromion is often referred to as the suprahumeral space and includes several soft tissues which can be "pinched" if inadequate muscular action, decreased space, or enlargement of soft tissues occurs. This is typically described as classic impingement syndrome and should be defined as specifically as possible to enable definitive care. There are some individuals who may have a higher susceptibility to this condition related to bony encroachment. (Nicholson et al., 1996).

SHOULDER: STANDARD PLAIN RADIOGRAPHS

The initial screening views of the glenohumeral joint traditionally begin with the antero-posterior (AP) external rotation (supine with external rotation of the humerus, palm up) and AP internal rotation (supine with forearm and palm down across abdomen) (Figures 5–2 and 5–3). In external rotation, the greater tuberosity is in profile as the most lateral projection. While in internal rotation, the lesser tuberosity is in profile on the medial aspect of the humeral head against the glenoid. These views give an overall appreciation of the proximal portion of the humerus, the lateral aspects of the clavicle, and the acromioclavicular (AC) joint as well as the upper portions of the scapula (Greathouse, 1998).

Clavicle and AC joint assessment is accomplished via a standing bilateral AP image. Clavicle fractures are typically revealed adequately with conventional radiography (Figure 5–4). If AC separation is suspected, a weighted view is performed with weight suspended from the wrist on the affected side. The examiner measures the

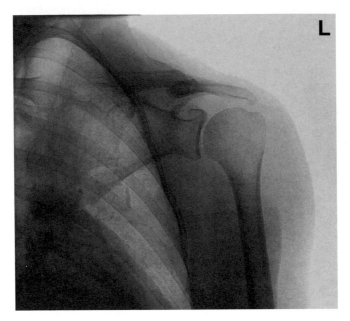

Figure 5–2 In this AP radiograph, the humerus is positioned in external rotation as indicated by the prominence of the greater tuberosity laterally.

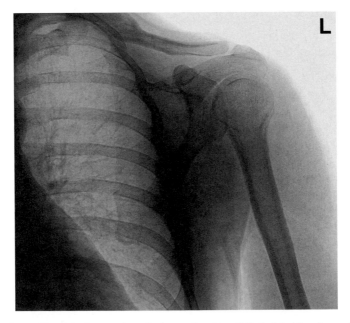

Figure 5–3 The profile of the lesser tuberosity is prominent medially in this AP radiograph, consistent with an internally rotated position.

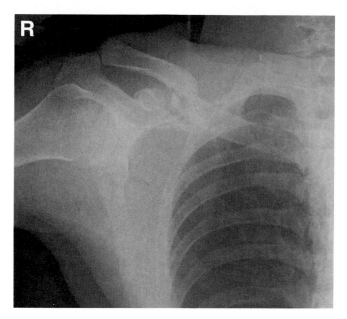

Figure 5–4 In this radiograph, a fracture of the middle third of the clavicle is evident. Owing to the angle of the middle third and superimposition, fractures in this region may be more difficult to visualize than those more proximal or distal.

amount of clavicle elevation and widening of the joint proper in these two views (Figures 5–5A & B).

Scapular screening includes the AP and lateral views. The AP view typically is performed supine with the upper extremity in the 90–90 position (90 degrees of abduction and 90 degrees of external rotation), enabling the scapular borders and angles to be

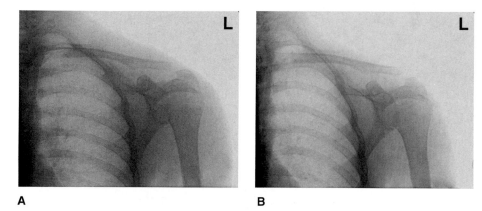

A **B**

Figure 5–5 A. Widening of the space between the distal clavicle and proximal acromion is evident in this AP radiograph, consistent with ligamentous injury. **B.** This space is enhanced with suspension of weight from the patient's upper extremity, further highlighting the ligamentous injury.

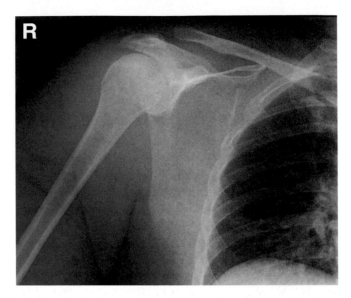

Figure 5–6 The fracture lines in the scapula are difficult to visualize in this AP radiograph. The extent of fracture is actually severe enough to be considered as comminuted. CT is often superior for identifying and delineating scapular fractures.

outlined and thus evaluated (Figure 5–6). The lateral view permits the body of the scapula to be seen most clearly as the ribs are not in a superimposed projection. Humerus screening requires an AP and lateral view if fracture assessment is suspected. Proximal fractures of the humerus are often classified by specific location within the bone: described as greater or lesser tuberosity, head, or surgical neck fractures (see Figure 5–1). Displacement forms the second portion of the indexing as these fractures are either displaced or nondisplaced. Fortunately, the majority of proximal humerus fractures are nondisplaced and can be treated rather effectively with conservative measures. (Figures 5–7 and 5–8). Radiography may also be adequate for identifying greater tuberosity fractures, although computed tomography (CT) may be required (Figure 5–9).

Alternative or specialized views are sometimes used in an attempt to better define specific structures often following trauma or injury. A good example is the evaluation of patients who have sustained a shoulder dislocation. The West Point or Lawrence View (inferior-superior axial projection) attempts to display the inferior glenoid fossa and its relationship to the humeral head (Figure 5–10) as well as the lateral perspective of the proximal humerus—sometimes demonstrating a Bankart lesion/fracture, particularly following an anterior-inferior glenohumeral shoulder dislocation (a bony separation at the glenoid edge) (Figures 5–11 and 5–12). A "sister lesion" is sometimes present on the posterior-lateral humeral head where it impacts the glenoid as the dislocation occurs (Figure 5–13). This scuffing injury, often referred to as a Hill-Sachs lesion, to the humerus can become quite large in the patient with numerous recurrent dislocations.

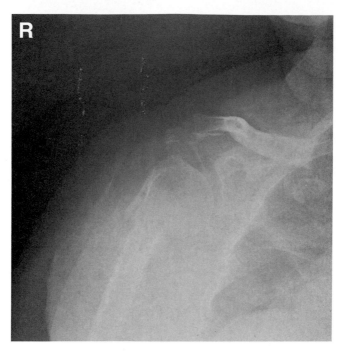

Figure 5–7 In this AP radiograph, a fracture of the neck of the humerus is evident. Note the malalignment of the fracture fragments. Also observe the fracture line is less defined, suggesting some early healing.

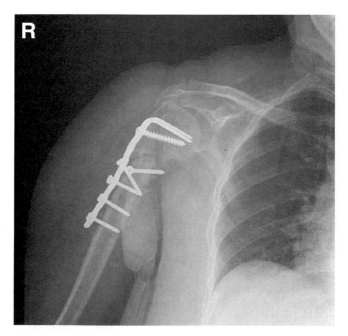

Figure 5–8 In this later radiograph of the same patient as in Figure 5–7 after undergoing open reduction internal fixation, complications with the hardware are visible. Note separation of the plate from the cortex distally and the retraction of the screws.

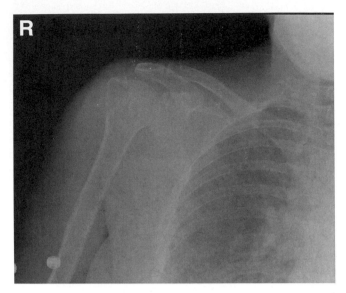

Figure 5–9 The findings are subtle on this image, but close inspection reveals a fracture of the greater tuberosity.

A scapular Y lateral (anterior oblique projection) is often used when there is a clinical presentation of trauma possibly associated with fractures of the scapula or proximal humerus. This view provides a Y appearance through the acromion and coracoid projecting vertically atop the scapular body. These special views are again typically used when specific trauma provides a suspicion of a particular injury or

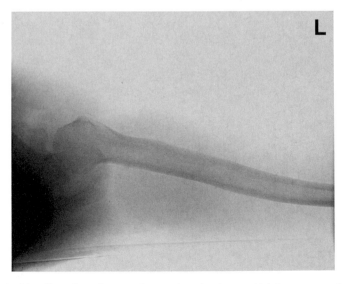

Figure 5–10 In this axillary view of a normal-appearing glenohumeral joint, a more precise assessment can be gained of the relationship between the humeral head and the glenoid fossa.

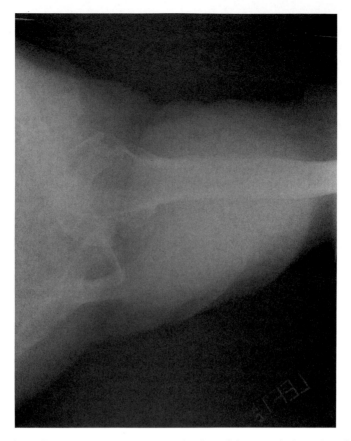

Figure 5–11 This axillary view demonstrates a complete loss of the normal relationship of the humeral head and glenoid fossa, typical of a frank dislocation.

when the patient is unable to assume some of the other traditional radiographic positions.

As the case in other regions, radiography is often adequate to demonstrate progressing degenerative changes. Radiographic findings of AC joint degeneration often include hypertrophy of the distal clavicle and proximal acromion (Figure 5–14). Among the degenerative changes typical of the shoulder include a loss of glenohumeral joint space and osteophyte formation at the tip of the acromion (Figure 5–15). Degenerative changes within the rotator cuff and other soft tissue structures are best demonstrated with MRI.

Owing to the overlapping layers of osseous tissues and superimposition on radiographs, CT is often undertaken when the index of suspicion for possible fractures is particularly elevated. Delineation of fracture extent and fragment location with CT is particularly superior to radiography (Figures 5–16 to 5–18).

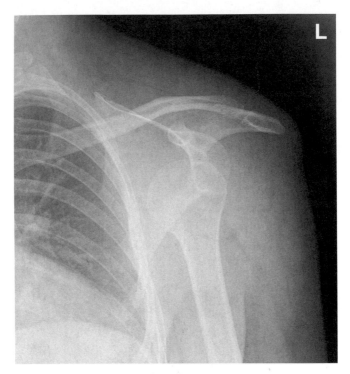

Figure 5–12 This AP radiograph clearly reveals anterior-inferior dislocation of the humeral head. Often the clinical signs are so obvious that radiographs are not completed until reduction has been attempted and imaging is completed to assess postreduction alignment.

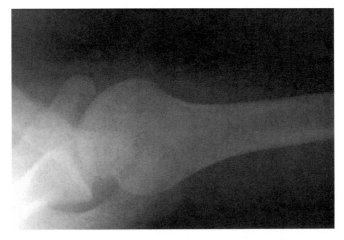

Figure 5–13 This axillary view radiograph reveals a tell-tale deformity of the posterior humeral head known as a Hill-Sachs lesion. This deformity accompanies glenohumeral dislocations as the humeral head is compressed and abraded against the edge of the glenoid fossa, resulting in an indentation of the humeral head.

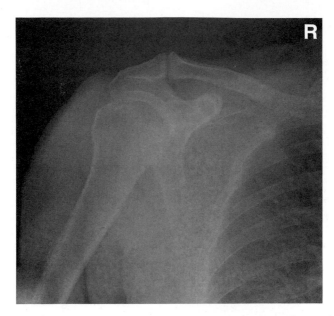

Figure 5–14 Enlargement of the articular surfaces of the AC joint are evident in this radiograph, which is typical of degenerative change.

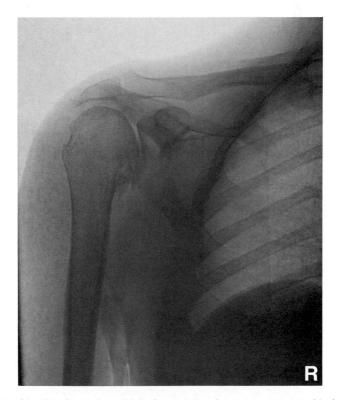

Figure 5–15 In this AP radiograph, multiple degenerative changes are suggested including the loss of glenohumeral joint space, hypertrophy of the AC joint, and osteophyte formation at the tip of the acromion.

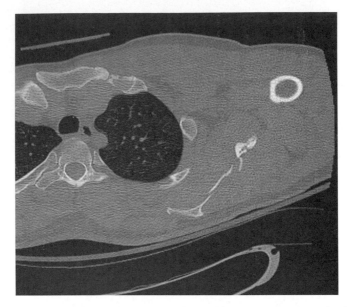

Figure 5–16 In this axial view CT, a comminuted fracture of the scapula is evident. The detail provided by CT is superior to radiography for such suspected injuries. For greater description and discussion of this process, see the enclosed instructional CD.

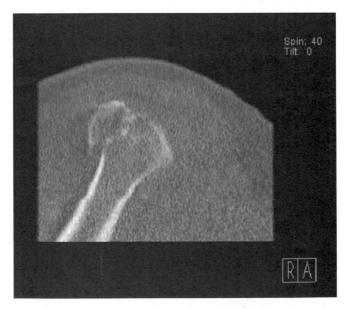

Figure 5–17 In this CT image, fracture of the greater tuberosity is evident. Note the markers on the image indicating the right side and from an anterior perspective.

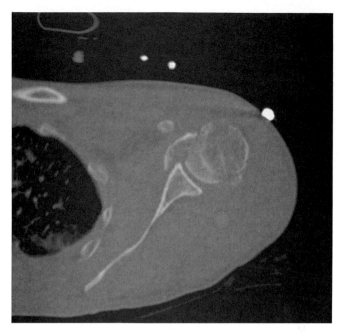

Figure 5–18 In this axial view CT, multiple fragments comprising the humeral head are evident. Thus, CT can not only assist in identifying the fracture, but provide detail concerning the fragments not possible on radiography.

 ## SOFT TISSUE STRUCTURES OF THE SHOULDER

One of the greatest challenges to the clinician related to shoulder imaging is to gain an appreciation of the numerous soft tissues which either move or control both actively and passively the shoulder complex. These capsular ligaments and muscle–tendon units are vital to normal shoulder function and will be discussed respectively. The capsule is composed of fibrous collagen tissues with either a loose pattern or well-defined bundles to provide stability particularly at end ranges of motion. The capsule inserts to the glenoid through the fibrocartilagenous labrum. This leads to a common problem associated with shoulder dislocations as the capsule is unable to reattach to the underlying glenoid as the labrum has insufficient vascularity to support healing. The classic tear is anterior-inferior and is called a Bankart lesion, and if it includes a glenoid bony separation, it is called a Bankart fracture. Traditionally, the radiologist used an arthrogram to demonstrate these lesions, but today MRI and its greater specificity has supplanted the earlier techniques (Figure 5–19). CT is still used for suspected fractures, particularly of the glenoid rim.

Another set of ligaments includes the AC ligaments and the coracoclavicular ligaments. The AC ligaments are responsible for AP stability, while the coracoclavicular ligaments control vertical displacement of the clavicle. Vertical instability is documented via plain films, especially a weighted view as displayed in Figure 5–5.

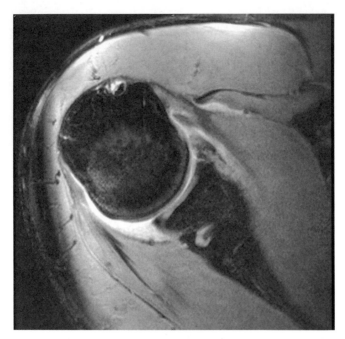

Figure 5–19 This axial slice MRI reveals multiple significant findings. The anterior capsulolabral structures demonstrate substantial discontinuity. The additional finding of indentation of the posterior humeral head is consistent with a Hill-Sachs lesion with accompanying subjacent marrow edema. These suggest the glenohumeral joint had been dislocated.

The muscle–tendon units are often the unhappy occupants of a constrained space which has the tendency for compression and thus increasing the likelihood of tendon damage. The most commonly affected tendon is the supraspinatus (as part of the rotator cuff), and complete and incomplete injuries are seen. The traditional mode of imaging was the arthrogram, particularly with a contrast agent to better fill or delineate defects. Today, both MRI and ultrasound are being used with greater sensitivity and specificity. Real-time ultrasound perhaps holds promise as both a clinical and assessment imaging device to facilitate instruction in muscular actions along with documenting tendon composition (Figure 5–20). The capacity of MRI to detect changes in tissues is demonstrated readily with imaging of the rotator cuff as the range of tissue changes from subtle age-related changes to frank tears (Figures 5–21 to 5–23). Bursal tissues can be imaged through contrast arthrography, but this is not done on a regular basis as the loss of motion seen in association with capsular adhesions or restrictions is delineated efficiently via clinical presentation.

Labral pathology is another tissue which can require radiographic assessment. Since the labrum is fibrocartilagenous, special techniques are used including contrast arthrography and MRI. Labral problems are frequently either superior (superior labrum anterior to posterior [SLAP]) or inferior (Bankart lesion). These both are often linked to underlying capsular instability and are then a concomitant finding for the patient being evaluated related to a recent dislocation. The SLAP patient is typically a 20- to 40-year-old

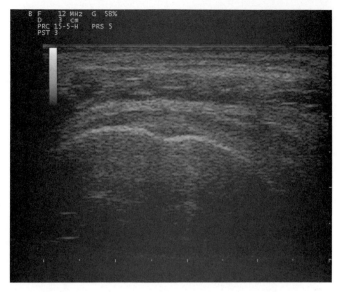

Figure 5–20 This ultrasonographic image of a normal-appearing supraspinatus muscle and tendon demonstrates consistent echogenicity in the tissue and the fascial planes outlining the muscle are continuous.

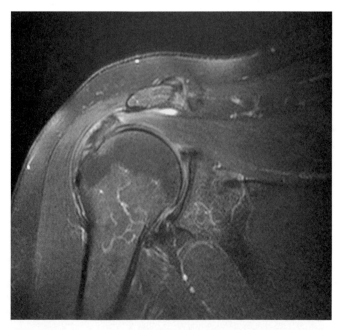

Figure 5–21 In this coronal slice MRI, note the outline of the supraspinatus suggests continuity, but with heterogeneous signal intensity. Such change in signal intensity is consistent with inflammation (increased signal) and degeneration (decreased signal).

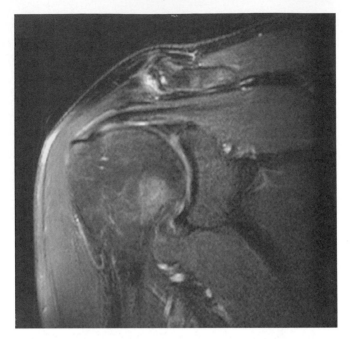

Figure 5–22 In this coronal slice MRI, note the change in signal intensity within the supraspinatus tendon. This most likely represents a partial-thickness tear. Concurrently on this image, note the increased signal intensity at the AC joint, which is consistent with inflammatory response.

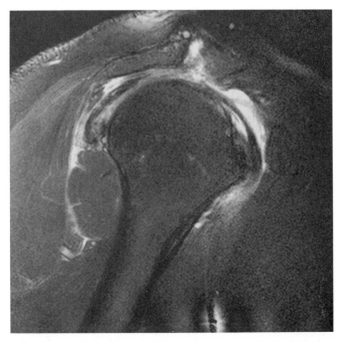

Figure 5–23 This sagittal slice MRI demonstrates a massive tear of the rotator cuff. Note the lack of continuity of the supraspinatus tendon accompanying the inflammatory response.

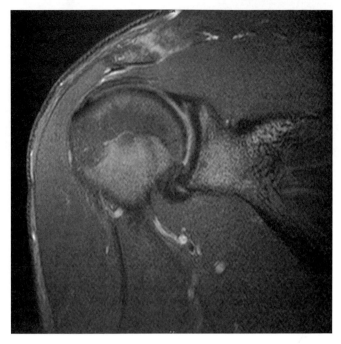

Figure 5–24 The superior portion of the labrum is suggested to be discontinuous in this coronal slice MRI. This is likely to represent a SLAP lesion.

male with a history of overhand throwing (Figure 5–24). Still greater sensitivity in examining the labrum can be achieved by the addition of injected contrast into the joint with a MR arthrogram (Figures 5–25A & B). The benefit of greater sensitivity occurring from the capsulolabral structures being distended in addition to the contrast allowing increased definition of the structures.

Occasionally, imaging will identify incidental findings which may or may not be of relevance for the particular clinical presentations of interest (Figure 5–26).

 ## CLINICAL RELEVANCE TO PHYSICAL THERAPY

Rehabilitation Implications

An important point is that the superior labrum has numerous normal variations or orientations of insertion onto the glenoid. SLAP lesions have become a more visible entity through the emergence of MRI. Just as at the knee, the MRI has provided much greater ability for the clinician to appreciate pathology in a variety of tissues. Interestingly, surgeons must recognize that the numerous variations of insertion of the labrum should not be read/interpreted as pathologic but recognized as a normal variant. This same process has evolved at the knee where previously read meniscal tears are now described as altered signal—consistent with changes but not always labeled as a tear through to the surface of the meniscus.

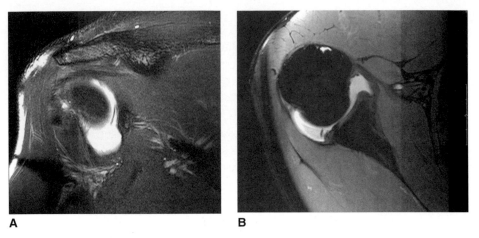

A   **B**

Figure 5–25 A. With distention of the capsule from injected contrast agent, this MR arthrogram delineates a posterior labral lesion well. In this axial view, observe the projection from the posterior labrum consistent with fraying and possible cumulative trauma. In this coronal image, note the frayed and detached edge of the labrum. **B.** In this axial view of the same patient, observe the projection from the posterior labrum consistent with fraying and possible cumulative trauma.

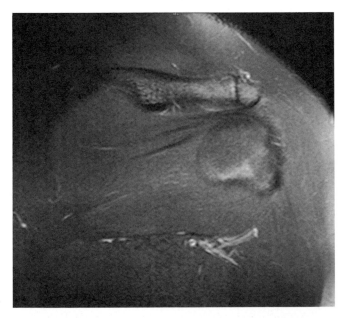

Figure 5–26 In this coronal slice MRI of the left shoulder, an os acromiale (non-union or incomplete fusion of the acromion) is revealed. This finding may be incidental, or may have direct clinical applicability as in this case for the patient presenting with an impingement syndrome.

A 28-year-old softball player reported to the clinic with complaints of catching and popping of his right shoulder. He had been a baseball pitcher from ages 9 to 22 and had become a traveling softball player the last several years. He exhibited 140 degrees of external rotation and only 40 degrees on internal rotation at the glenohumeral joint. He had a slight increase in anterior and posterior capsular laxity. He had two positive impingement tests (Hawkin's and Elevation) and also was quite uncomfortable with the O'Brien's test in internal rotation but less tender with external rotation (again pointing toward labral pathology but being appreciative of possible underlying microinstability associated with throwing) (see Figure 5–24). So this type of athlete may present with superior labral pathology from the long-time history of overhead throwing (throwing athletes often have abnormal labral signal, which is very common in college and major league pitchers); abnormal signal associated with abrasion and tearing from the underlying microinstability; or as a normal variant. Fortunately, he did well with a rehabilitation program and was able to control his symptoms and continue to play softball several times on a weekly basis.

ADDITIONAL READING

Anderson, J. (2000). *An Atlas of radiography for sports injuries.* New York: McGraw-Hill.

Anderson, J., Read, J.W., & Steinweg, J. (2007). *Atlas of imaging in sports medicine.* New York: McGraw-Hill.

REFERENCES

Greathouse, J. (1998). *Radiographic positioning procedure.* Vol. 1.New York:Delmar Publishers.

Nicholson, G. P., Goodman, D. A., Flatow, E. L., & Bigliani, L. U. (1996). The acromion: Morphologic condition and age related changes. A study of 420 scapulas. *Shoulder and Elbow Surgery, 5,* 1–11.

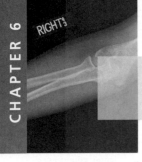

CHAPTER 6

The Elbow

Imaging of the elbow includes assessment of the three-joint complex: humeroulnar, humeroradial, and proximal radioulnar. The function of these three joints is to allow the hand to be positioned to enable the desired actions to be accomplished. The distal humerus provides medial (trochlea—articulates with ulna) and lateral (capitulum or capitellum—articulates with radius) articular areas of their respective condyles (Figure 6–1). Three concavities (fossae) are present, two anteriorly—coronoid (accepts/articulates with ulna in flexion) and radial (accepts/articulates with radius in flexion), while there is one posteriorly—olecranon (accepts/articulates with the olecranon process of the ulna in extension). The most proximal radius is composed of the head, which includes a cup-like superior projection to articulate with the capitulum, while the circumferential surface articulates with the radial notch of the ulna. The remaining proximal radius is composed of the bicipital tuberosity and the neck. The medial and lateral epicondyles of the humerus serve as insertional sites for ligaments and tendons.

ELBOW: RADIOGRAPHS

The minimal screening series for the elbow includes the anteroposterior (AP) and lateral projections. In some facilities, the additional oblique view is a part of protocol. Most of the time, elbow films are performed after trauma, and thus the focus is on fracture recognition, and often the forearm is also a part of the assessment related to the inter-relatedness of these functional units (Greathouse, 1998).

The AP view is taken with the patient seated and the elbow extended, externally rotated, and with the normal carrying angle (typically 10 to 15 degrees) of the individual. The film exhibits the distal humerus, proximal radius, proximal ulna, and their respective articulations (Figure 6–2). The general anatomy is relatively well defined with some superimposition of a portion of the radial head and proximal radius with ulna with the olecranon process of the ulna well seated on the trochlea and into the olecranon fossa, again superimposed through the humerus.

The lateral view is accomplished with the patient seated and the elbow flexed to 90 degrees and the thumb up (neutral forearm position). This view best outlines the olecranon and the anterior radial head in profile. It also can exhibit supracondylar humerus fractures, particularly through the fat pad sign—soft tissue projections (fat pad) out of their normal fossa locations (Figure 6–3).

Oblique views are sometimes added if concern is focused on the coronoid process (internal oblique rotation view) or the proximal radius/head (external oblique rotation view).

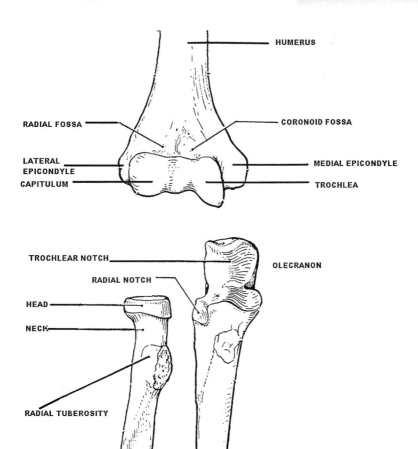

Figure 6–1 Diagram of bony features of the elbow.

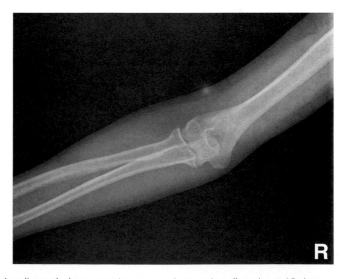

Figure 6–2 A radiograph demonstrating a normal-appearing elbow in an AP view.

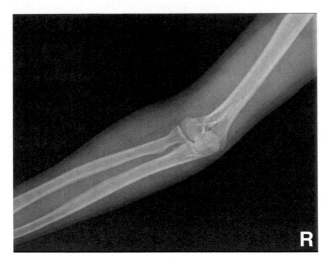

Figure 6–3 A lateral view radiograph of a normal-appearing elbow.

These structures are not superimposed and are thus in profile through these rotations. The patient is seated as in the other standard views during this radiograph.

Clinicians may need to alter these projections if there is a limitation of elbow extension or other motion limitations not allowing the patient to be positioned as described. Likewise, to allow very specific structural delineation, films may be done such as a full (acute) flexion view to profile the olecranon process (patient seated and the elbow flexed maximally).

The forearm is typically assessed through AP and lateral views. The AP radiograph is performed with the patient seated, elbow extended, and the palm upward, while the lateral radiograph is accomplished with the patient seated, elbow flexed, and the thumb upward (neutral wrist position) (Figure 6–4). The numerous types and descriptions as well as radiographic appearances of forearm fractures are provided in Chapter 7.

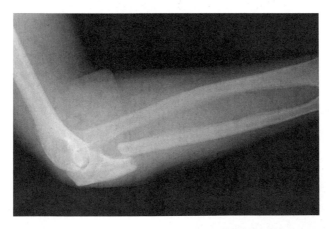

Figure 6–4 A fracture with considerable displacement of the proximal ulna is demonstrated in this lateral view radiograph.

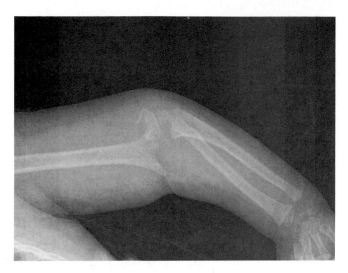

Figure 6–5 In this radiograph, a fracture dislocation of the elbow is demonstrated in a 3-year-old. The fracture evident on this image is consistent with a Salter-Harris type I epiphyseal fracture.

Proximal and distal humeral fractures commonly occur associated with falls, often described as a FOOSH (fall on an outstretched hand) injury. The distal injuries are often categorized as to anatomic location of the fracture line. When the fracture line is above the condyles but not into the normal shaft, the term is *supracondylar* and is very common in children but rare in adults (Figures 6–5 and 6–6A & B). Since most falls occur

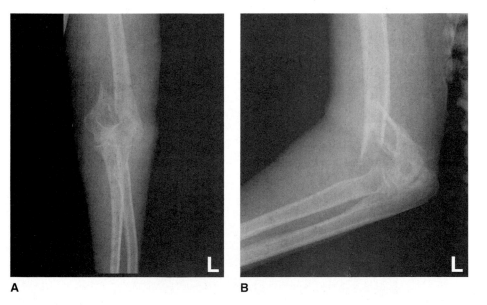

A   B

Figure 6–6 These AP (A) and lateral (B) radiographs demonstrate a supracondylar fracture with displacement. Considering the displacement present from these views and the proximity to critical peripheral nerves and blood vessels, one can easily understand the potential for neurovascular involvement with such fractures.

with elbow extension, the child displaces the distal humerus posteriorly, placing neurovascular structures at risk.

Fractures through the condyles are known as transcondylar fractures, while those that go through the condyles and also split them into medial and lateral fragments are referred to as intercondylar fractures and are sometimes called Y or T fractures associated with their radiographic appearance. This intercondylar fracture is the most frequently seen fracture of the distal humerus in adults in contrast to children. One of the great concerns with children is growth plate closure and this is sometimes seen when a single condyle is fractured—typically known as a condylar fracture. These fractures are again rare in adults but somewhat common in children. These fractures are typically well displayed via the standard screen views (AP, lateral, and oblique if used). When articular surfaces are involved, computed tomography (CT) imaging is sometimes employed to better delineate surface detail (Figure 6–7). CT is also valuable for fully delineating other bony abnormalities in and around the joint. One such phenomenon occasionally occurring at the elbow is heterotopic ossification (Figures 6–8A & B).

Radial head fractures are classified by displacement and fragmentation. Type I is a nondisplaced single fragment, type II is a displaced single fragment, and type III is comminuted (multiple fragments) often associated radial head resection as the treatment technique with some increasing use of prosthetic head replacements in younger patients. Type I injuries are nearly always treated nonoperatively through immobilization and relatively rapid functionalization. The type II injuries are more challenging, and treatment varies from immobilization to resection based on level of displacement and patient

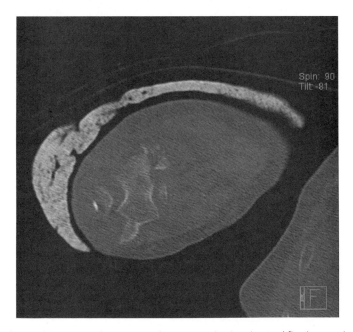

Figure 6–7 This axial CT image of the elbow after open reduction–internal fixation continues to reveal significant bone fragmentation. CT, with multiple views, allows better understanding of the fragment size and location.

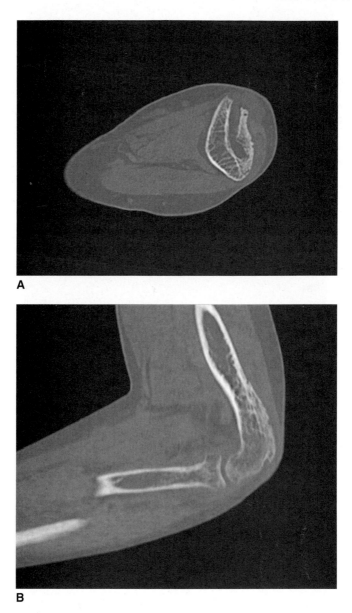

A

B

Figure 6–8 A. This axial CT image of the distal humerus at approximately the level of the epicondyles reveals a large area of heterotopic ossification posteriorly. **B.** This sagittal CT image of the elbow further delineates the size of the heterotopic ossification at the posterior aspect of the distal humerus.

response. Often radial head fractures are difficult to detect in the absence of displacement and may be indicated by the joint effusion causing fat pad prominence and a so-called "fat pad sign" on a lateral view radiograph (Figure 6–9).

Olecranon fractures are classified much like radial head injuries: displacement and fragmentation. The typical injury is caused by a fall onto the elbow with the resultant image revealing a fracture line which separates a distal fragment from the remaining olecranon. If

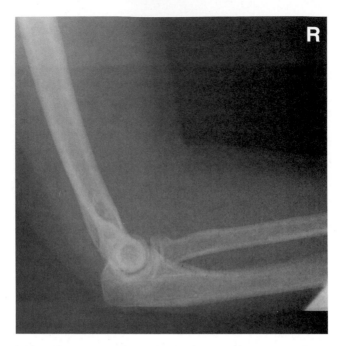

Figure 6–9 Radial head fractures are often difficult to detect as frank cortical disruption may not be evident. In this lateral view radiograph, a subtle finding such as the appearance of the anterior fat pad suggests an occult radial head fracture.

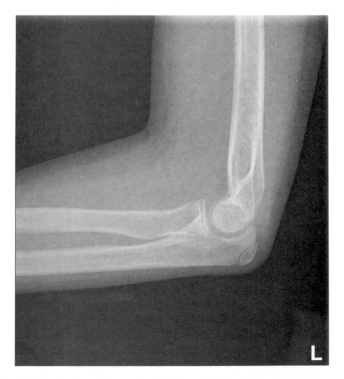

Figure 6–10 In this lateral view radiograph, a fracture of the tip of the olecranon process is evident.

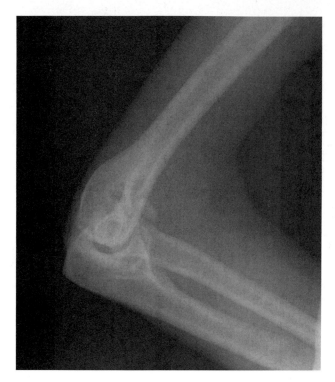

Figure 6–11 In this lateral view radiograph, the proximal ulna and radius structures are superimposed, making visualization of the radial head fracture difficult. The coronoid process fracture is more evident. Fractures of this structure are common with subluxations and dislocations.

nondisplaced, nonoperative treatment is the rule, whereas open reduction internal fixation is typical of displaced fractures. The traditional screen plain films are sufficient for these injuries other than when the anterior coronoid process fractures are suspected (as with a posterior elbow dislocation) when an oblique view is added to the screen (Figures 6–10 and 6–11).

Elbow dislocations are fortunately rare but are seen in response to a fall and other direct trauma. The most common is to have posterior displacement of the ulna and radius posteriorly on the humerus. Reduction can be difficult and sometimes requires anesthetic agents. The typical screen views are successful in delineating this injury (Figure 6–12).

As radiography is typically adequate to allow appropriate clinical decision making, magnetic resonance imaging (MRI) is utilized with relative infrequency about the elbow, but may be used to investigate soft tissue injuries (Figure 6–13).

 ## CLINICAL RELEVANCE TO PHYSICAL THERAPY

Rehabilitation Implications

A 16-year-old high school pitcher presented to the clinic with the complaint of progressive "elbow pain" associated with playing baseball and pitching in particular. His pain had forced him not to pitch the last 10 days, and his pain was primarily localized to the

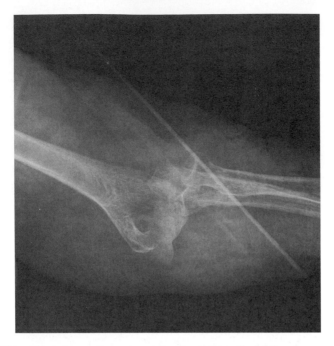

Figure 6–12 This oblique view radiograph reveals a frank dislocation of the elbow.

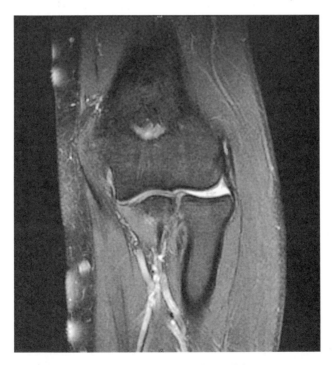

Figure 6–13 This coronal plane MR image reveals a partial tear of the common extensor tendon from the lateral epicondyle. This is indicated by the increased signal intensity at the area. Also note the neighboring fluid signal within the radiohumeral joint.

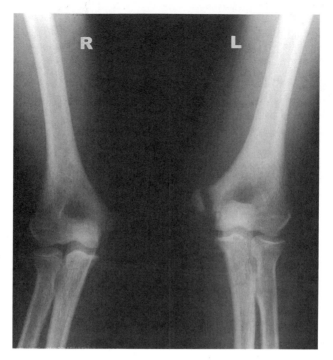

Figure 6–14 These two images, comparing sides in a skeletally immature male, reveal an avulsion fracture of the left medial epicondyle. These injuries are frequently observed in young throwing athletes.

medial epicondyle. The AP image (Figure 6–14) clearly demonstrates the altered appearance of the medial epicondyle. This is in response to the high medial strain loads seen during pitching. It is estimated that the average high school pitcher threw more than 1,000,000 "throws" in the development of the mature pitching motion. This presentation is the final outcome of what often begins as Little League elbow and is very much an overload upon the skeletally immature athlete. We have seen a significant increase in this patient presentation as athletes are specializing in a single sport at earlier ages and also participate year round rather than in a single season.

ADDITIONAL READING

Anderson, J. (2000). *An Atlas of radiography for sports injuries.* New York: McGraw-Hill.

Anderson, J., Read, J.W., & Steinweg, J. (2007). *Atlas of imaging in sports medicine.* New York: McGraw-Hill.

REFERENCE

Greathouse, J. (1998). *Radiographic positioning procedure.* Vol. 1. Delmar Publishers. New York: Albany.

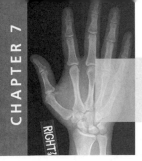
Imaging of the Forearm, Wrist, and Hand

In the forearm, reference to normal anatomic relationships begins with the radius and ulna, proximal to distal. The distal radioulnar joint is a critical articulation in forearm pronation and supination. This joint has a separate synovial compartment and bordered distally by the triangular fibrocartilage (May, 2002). Generally, the radial styloid process extends beyond the ulnar styloid process by approximately 9 to 12 mm. At the proximal articular surface of the lunate, however, the two bones are of approximately of the same level. An ulna of less length provides for negative ulnar variance, and a longer ulna is described by a positive ulnar variance. The normal arrangement of the distal ulna and radius provides for the radial angle (also known as the ulnar slant or ulnar inclination), which is usually measured at 15 to 25 degrees. The distal surface of the radius also demonstrates an orientation toward the palmar or volar surface of approximately 10 to 25 degrees (Greenspan, 2000; May, 2002). These anatomic relationships are critical in imaging assessment for the orthopedist, both in assessing for pathology and in planning the appropriate course of intervention (Figures 7–1 and 7–2).

At the articular surface of the ulna is the triangular fibrocartilage complex (TFCC), which functionally extends the distal ulna to be approximately the same length of the radius. The TFCC consists of the triangular fibrocartilage, dorsal and volar radioulnar ligaments, sheath of the extensor carpi ulnaris tendon, ulnocarpal ligaments, ulnar collateral ligament, and ulnomeniscal homologue. Of significance is the triangular fibrocartilage's tendency to be thicker peripherally and it may attenuate centrally to have a small opening. In addition to contributing to stability of the wrist, the TFCC also provides for a cushion between the proximal carpals and distal radius. The proximal row of carpals, forming an arc, consists of the scaphoid, lunate, and triquetrum, connected by their interosseous ligaments. The pisiform is also included in the proximal row, but as a sesamoid bone is more loosely connected than the others and is located in the flexor carpi ulnaris tendon anterior to the triquetrum. Another anatomic alignment consideration is the palmar orientation of the scaphoid of approximately 45 degrees. This proximal row functions as a linkage between the distal radius and the distal row of carpals. The distal row of the trapezium, trapezoid, capitate, and hamate also forms an arc in articulating with the bases of the metacarpals. The lunate and capitate form a central carpal column, which is functionally important for force transmission. The concave volar surface of the carpals, covered by the wrist joint capsule, forms the dorsal boundary of the carpal tunnel. The volar border of the carpal tunnel is the flexor retinaculum. Contained in the tunnel are the flexor tendons and median nerve, passing through to their distal endpoints in the hand. The other fibro-osseous tunnel-like structure on the

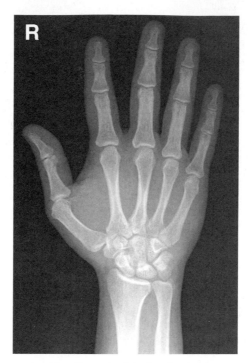

Figure 7–1 A normal-appearing PA radiograph of the hand and wrist.

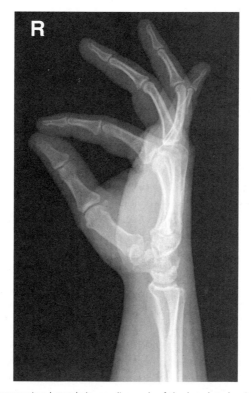

Figure 7–2 A normal-appearing lateral view radiograph of the hand and wrist.

volar aspect of the wrist is the tunnel of Guyon, containing the ulnar nerve and accompanying artery and vein. Of the volar and dorsal capsular ligaments of the wrist, the volar are generally stronger, although both are critical to wrist stability (May, 2002; Farooki et al., 2003).

On the dorsum of the wrist extending onto the hand and eventually to the digits are the extensor tendons, which are surrounded by synovial sheaths in six compartments. From a posterior to anterior view, the carpometacarpal joints normally have a "zig-zag" pattern. The first metacarpal articulates with the trapezium to form the first carpometacarpal joint. The second metacarpal articulates with the trapezoid, capitate, and the third metacarpal. The third metacarpal also articulates with the capitate. The fourth and fifth metacarpals articulate with the hamate. The third through fifth metacarpals are of decreasing length. All metacarpals articulate with the proximal phalanges, providing a course for the flexor tendons in synovial sheaths contained by fibro-osseous tunnels to their distal phalangeal attachments (May, 2002; Farooki et al., 2003).

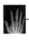 RADIOGRAPHY

In assessing the forearm, radiography is usually adequate to study the anatomic relationships of the radius and ulna. In basic posterior to anterior and lateral radiographs of the forearm and wrist, observation commonly begins with assessment of the normal anatomic relationships of the radius and ulna as described above.

A Monteggia's fracture–dislocation is the combination of dislocation of the radial head along with a fracture of the proximal ulnar shaft. Four variants of this have been described but the basic description applies in the majority of cases. This injury typically occurs from forced pronation during a fall or a direct impact on the posterior ulna (Greenspan, 2000; May 2002) (Figure 7–3).

The classic Galeazzi's fracture–dislocation consists of a fracture of the distal shaft of the radius with considerable displacement or angulation. The distal ulna is dislocated, most often in a dorsal and medial orientation. Thus, the distal radioulnar joint is dislocated, which may lead to chronic instability. Because of the complexity of the injury additional radiographic views or additional imaging modalities may be required (May, 2002; Resnick, 2000; Greenspan, 2000) (Figure 7–4).

Fractures of the distal radius are very common with multiple classification systems beyond the scope of this book. Several eponyms have been applied to various distal radius fractures and remain well engrained in clinical practice. Most frequently, these injuries occur among women over age 40 with osteoporosis, typically due to a fall onto an outstretched hand. These injuries may also occur in younger patients, but usually from high-energy trauma (Goldfarb et al., 2001; Resnick, 2000).

Perhaps most common is the Colles' fracture, which typically occurs from a fall on an outstretched hand while the forearm is pronated and the wrist extended (Goldfarb, 2001; Greenspan, 2000). By Colles' classic description, this is a transverse fracture of the distal radial metaphyseal area with dorsal angulation and displacement of the distal fragment (Colles, 1972). Comminution is common and there may be associated injuries

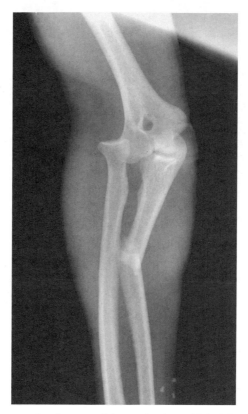

Figure 7–3 This PA view reveals a fracture of the proximal one-third of the ulna along with dislocation of the radial head, which is consistent with Monteggia's fracture.

such as ulnar styloid fracture, disruption of the distal radioulnar joint, and extension into the radiocarpal joint line (Greenspan, 2000; May, 2002). The deformity due to the dorsal angulation of the distal fragment has been described as being similar to an upside down fork (May, 2002). Important for the rehabilitation clinician is that Colles' fractures often heal with less than optimal alignment complicating recovery of function. Ulnar inclination and radial length are often lost as is volar tilt of the articular surface (May, 2002). Other complications include median nerve injury and eventual radiocarpal osteoarthritis (Greenspan, 2000; May, 2002) (Figure 7–5).

A Smith's fracture is a reversed Colles' fracture in which the fracture of the metaphyseal area demonstrates volar displacement and angulation of the distal fracture fragment. This injury is considerably less frequent than Colles' fractures. Most often, Smith's fractures occur in younger patients with high-energy trauma on a flexed wrist or a fall on the dorsum of the hand (Goldfarb et al., 2001; Greenspan, 2000; May, 2002) (Figure 7–6).

A Barton's fracture describes a shear-type fracture of the distal articular surface of the radius with translation of the distal radius fragment and accompanying dislocation or subluxation of the carpus. The classic Barton's fracture describes dorsal displacement, but a variant with volar displacement is referred to as a reverse Barton's fracture. Open

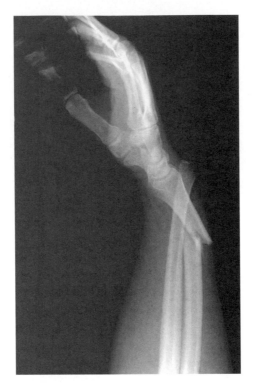

Figure 7–4 A lateral view radiograph demonstrating a fracture of the distal one-third of the radius along with dislocation of the distal radioulnar joint, which is often referred to as Galeazzi's fracture.

reduction and internal fixation are usually required (Goldfarb et al., 2001; Resnick, 2000; May, 2002) (Figure 7–7)..

Hutchinson's (chauffeur's) fracture consists of an oblique, intra-articular fracture of the distal radius. The radial styloid is within the fracture fragment along with the radial collateral ligament. The fracture fragment can vary considerably in size. These injuries often include associated intercarpal ligamentous injuries, especially of the scapholunate ligament. The mechanism of this fracture is usually a shear or translational injury with force transmitted through the scaphoid or scapholunate joint. Chauffeur's fractures were was named prior to the advent of electric starters on automobiles as the recoil on hand cranks were frequently the causative force (Goldfarb et al., 2001; Resnick, 2000; Greenspan, 2000; May, 2002) (Figure 7–8).

A die-punch fracture may include several different intra-articular fracture patterns, although it typically occurs in the lunate fossa of the distal radius. A transverse load transmitted through the lunate results in a depressed fracture of the articular surface of the distal radius. Comminution may occur and may not be adequately visualized on radiographs (Resnick, 2000; Goldfarb et al., 2001).

In assessing the wrist, the examiner looks for opposing articular surfaces to be aligned congruently, and a lack of this arrangement may suggest displacement of at least one of the articulating bones (Resnick, 2000; Greenspan, 2000). Intercarpal joint

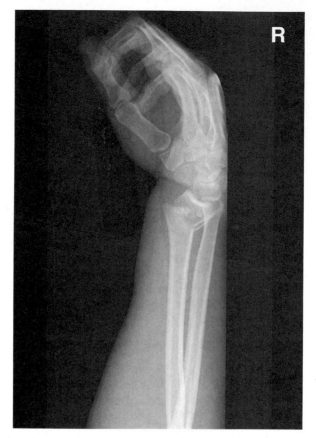

Figure 7–5 This lateral view radiograph reveals a Colles' fracture as defined by a transverse fracture line of the distal radius with dorsal angulation of the distal fragment.

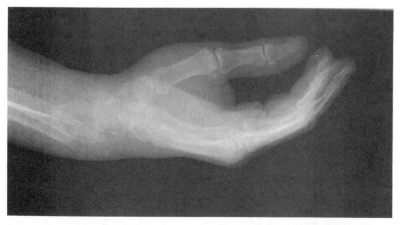

Figure 7–6 A radiograph view demonstrating the volar angulation of a distal radius fracture consistent with a Smith's fracture. In this image, close observation also reveals the ulnar styloid process also being fractured.

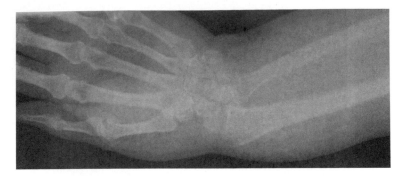

Figure 7–7 This PA view of the wrist reveals an intra-articular fracture of the distal radius along with dislocation of the proximal carpal row, known as a Barton's fracture.

spaces are normally equal and deviation from this evenness may be consistent with disruption of intercarpal ligamentous support and possible dislocation, pending the results of other views. Disturbance of these normal arcuate congruencies often occurs with fractures and dislocations. Multiple views of the wrist may be required to allow thorough examination of the carpals because of difficulty in visualizing fractures (Bohndorf and Kilcoyne, 2002; Goldfarb et al., 2001; Resnick, 2000). Scaphoid and triquetral

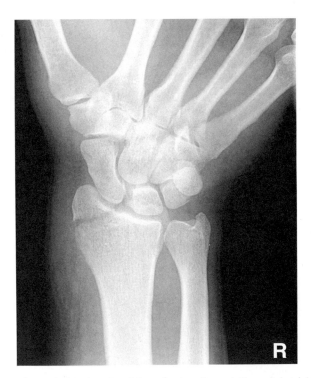

Figure 7–8 A PA radiograph showing the oblique fracture through the radial styloid process known as a Hutchinson's or chauffeur's fracture. *Image courtesy of Travis Fromwiller, MD, Department of Radiology, Medical College of Wisconsin, Milwaukee, Wisconsin.*

fractures are far more common than are fractures of the other carpal bones (Goldfarb et al., 2001). Fractures of the lunate and pisiform are relatively uncommmon. Fractures of the distal row of carpals are often associated with injury to the carpometacarapal joint (Resnick, 2000).

The scaphoid is the most frequent site of carpal fracture, accounting for 50 to 70 percent of all fractures involving the carpus. Most of these injuries occur at the waist and are nondisplaced (Farooki et al., 2003; Greenspan, 2000). In contrast to distal radius fractures, scaphoid fractures most frequently occur in young adults (May, 2002; Greenspan, 2000). The mechanism of injury is typically hyperextension of the wrist, but a pure compressive force can also result in fracture. The classic mechanism of falling on an outstretched hand causes palmar tensile and dorsal compressive force on the scaphoid (Goldfarb et al., 2001). Standard radiography is reported to detect 70 to 91 percent of scaphoid fractures (Leslie and Dickson, 1981; Brondum and Larsen, 1992; Fowler et al., 1998; Hauger et al., 2002; Moller et al., 2004). In addition to standard views, suspected scaphoid fractures may be imaged with the wrist in a position of ulnar deviation to provide further clarity (Goldfarb et al., 2001). A clenched fist may further sensitize the view for a fracture line (Bohndorf and Kilcoyne, 2002). Those fractures occurring across the waist and without displacement typically have good healing patterns, but those across the proximal pole may threaten the vascularity. The proximal portion of the bone has a particularly tenuous blood supply; thus, fracture with displacement increases the risk of avascular necrosis (Greenspan, 2000; May, 2002) (Figures 7–9 and 7–10).

The second most commonly fractured carpal bone is the triquetrum. Such fractures are best viewed by a lateral radiograph or a pronated oblique projection, demonstrating a small cortical fragment avulsed from the dorsal surface (Resnick, 2000; Greenspan,

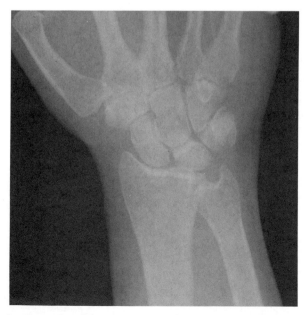

Figure 7–9 Only close inspection of the PA radiograph of the wrist suggests pathology of the scaphoid.

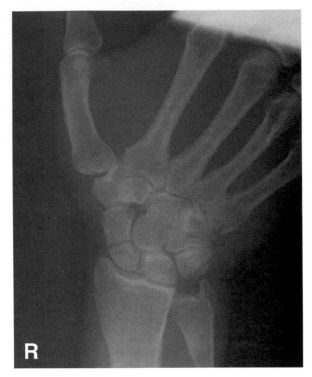

Figure 7–10 This image of the same patient as in Figure 7–9 repositioned in ulnar deviation clearly reveals the fracture line across the scaphoid. Similar effects are accomplished with the patient closing the hand into a fist or a tip-to-tip grasp of the first and second digits.

2000; May, 2002). Small chip avulsion fractures of the triquetrum may suggest associated ligamentous injury and may not be easily identified on radiographs owing to overlapping lucencies. Additional imaging may be required for differential diagnosis (Goldfarb et al., 2001; Greenspan, 2000) (Figure 7–11).

Fractures of the hook of the hamate typically occur from a direct blow to the volar aspect of the wrist. Often the recoil force of a golf club, baseball bat, racket, or a hammer may be the etiologic insult to injure the hook portion (May, 2002; Resnick, 2000; Greenspan, 2000; Goldfarb et al., 2001). The hook is usually visible on end with posteroanterior (PA) radiographs, appearing somewhat as if the letter "C" projects over the hamate. If displaced, the "C" may not be visible. A carpal tunnel view may be more revealing (May, 2002). Fractures also occur to the body of the hamate and are typically evident on lateral and pronated oblique standard projections (Greenspan, 2000). A dorsal articular fracture also occurs and may be accompanied by fourth and fifth carpometacarpal dislocations (Goldfarb et al., 2001).

Lunate fractures are unusual, but occur most frequently from a fall on an outstretched hand with extended wrist and a compressive mechanism (Greenspan, 2000). These injuries are often overlooked in the emergent setting because of difficulty in identifying the fractures on radiographs. The cortical lines of the neighboring carpus

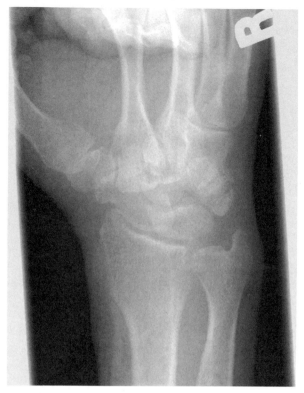

Figure 7–11 The oblique view radiograph reduces the overlapping lines of bone margins to reveal a fracture line through the triquetrum.

overlap the lunate, complicating identification (Goldfarb et al., 2001). PA and lateral projections are usually adequate to demonstrate this injury. Fractures often accompany perilunate dislocation and occur as a sequela to avascular necrosis (Kienböck's disease) (Greenspan, 2000) (Figure 7–12).

Kienböck's disease is avascular necrosis of the lunate and perhaps develops as a result of repeated trauma to the bone, resulting in collapse. On radiographs, the degenerating lunate may appear sclerotic and fragmented. (Goldfarb et al., 2001; Greenspan, 2000). A negative ulnar variance (as described in the anatomy introduction above) is associated with Kienböck's disease (Rosner, 2004) (Figure 7–13).

Fractures of the trapezium usually occur as a result of transverse loading with an adducted thumb as the first metacarpal is driven into the trapezium. Often these injuries are accompanied by other injuries to the first metacarpal and distal radius. Radiographs are typically adequate to diagnose the trapezium injury (Goldfarb et al., 2001). Trapezial ridge fractures are an exception, with particular difficulty in detection with plain films (Jayasekera et al., 2005).

Pisiform fractures often occur from a direct blow and may be difficult to detect on radiographs. Additionally, these injuries may occur in isolation, but usually occur with

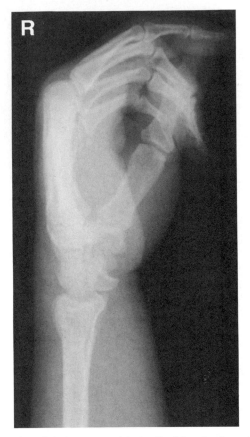

Figure 7–12 The malposition of the lunate consistent with dislocation is readily demonstrated in this lateral view radiograph.

other more obvious fractures, which may detract from their recognition. Nonunion or malunion are occasional complications (Goldfarb et al., 2001; Greenspan, 2000).

Capitate fractures are atypical and usually accompany other carpal injuries, such as scaphoid fracture or perilunate dislocation. Imaging beyond radiography is likely to be required to provide adequate detail (Goldfarb et al., 2001; Greenspan, 2000).

Trapezoid fractures are rarities in isolation owing to stable surrounding articulations (Jeong et al., 2001). Thus, if they occur, they may be accompanied by dislocation or dislocation of the second metacarpal. Radiographs are usually adequate for identification (Goldfarb et al., 2001).

A Bennett's fracture is an intra-articular fracture–dislocation at the first carpometacarpal joint. A small fragment of the base of the metacarpal remains in anatomic position in relation to the trapezium, while the metacarpal shaft is dislocated dorsoradially by the tension of the abductor pollicis longus muscle and tendon. Because of the instability, open reduction internal fixation is required. Radiography typically provides adequate viewing of this injury (Resnick, 2000; Greenspan, 2000; May, 2002) (Figure 7–14).

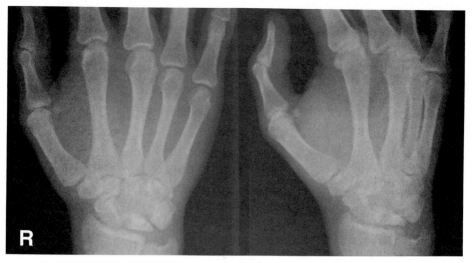

Figure 7–13 Collapse of the lunate is evident in these radiographs. Such appearance is consistent with Kienböck's disease.

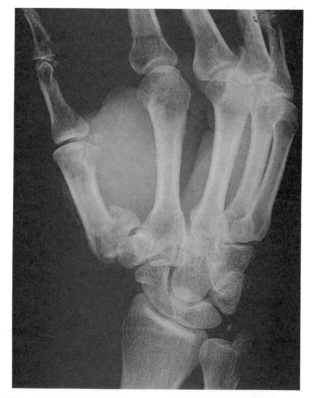

Figure 7–14 An oblique view radiograph demonstrating a Bennett's fracture at the proximal portion of the first phalanx. Note the dislocation of the metacarpal shaft from the proximal fracture fragment.
Image courtesy of Travis Fromwiller, MD, Department of Radiology, Medical College of Wisconsin, Milwaukee, Wisconsin.

Rolando's fracture is a Bennett's fracture with comminution in a T- or Y-shaped configuration of fracture lines at the metacarpal base. Because of the comminution, restoration of anatomic alignment is unlikely and open reduction with internal fixation (ORIF) of small fracture fragments is usually not possible. Thus, closed reduction is usually the chosen course of treatment. Owing to the potential for fragmentation of the base of the metacarpal, additional imaging may be required beyond radiography (Resnick, 2000; Greenspan, 2000; May, 2002) (Figure 7–15).

Fractures of the necks of the metacarpals are common. These injuries typically occur from an axial load on a clenched fist. Displacement of the bone ends is common with volar angulation of the distal fragment. Fracture lines may be spiral or oblique and cause overlap of the bone ends on radiographs (Resnick, 2000). The most common fracture involves the fifth metacarpal.

The term *boxer's fracture* has long been used to describe a fracture of the fifth metacarpal, usually from punching with a closed fist. Boxers, however, more frequently fracture the neck of their second or third metacarpals. Most cases of conventionally termed boxer's fractures are due to punching of inanimate objects with the dominant hand. The fracture is usually across the neck of the metacarpal with volar angulation of the distal fragment. Persistent deformity of angulation and foreshortening of the metacarpal is common (May, 2000; Greenspan, 2000; Brandser and Ellington, 2000). This injury will often be observed in males spanning adolescence through young adulthood (Figure 7–16).

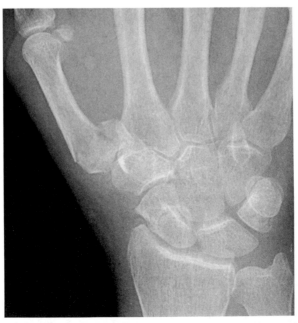

Figure 7–15 A Rolando's fracture is evident in this radiograph as a "T" fracture line configuration is present. *Image courtesy of Travis Fromwiller, MD, Department of Radiology, Medical College of Wisconsin, Milwaukee, Wisconsin.*

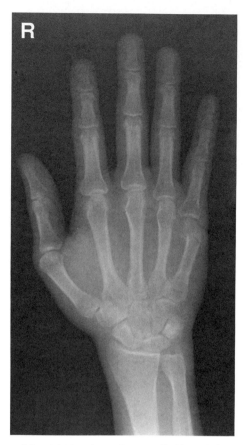

Figure 7–16 This PA view of the right hand reveals a so-called boxer's fracture with a fracture of the distal portion of the fifth metacarpal with volar angulation.

Ligamentous instability injuries are not directly visualized on radiographs, but rather will be implied by an obvious disruption in normal anatomic relationships. If these injuries are suspected, more sophisticated imaging is often completed to provide greater detail. Limited use of radiography, however, often precedes magnetic resonance imaging (MRI), computerized tomography (CT), or other imaging.

Disruption of the ulnar collateral ligament at the first metacarpophalangeal joint results in what is traditionally known as gamekeeper's thumb, arising from abduction stresses as gamekeepers sacrificed their animals. Such injuries now occur more often from forceful abduction mechanisms such as that from a ski pole or in break dancers. Avulsion of a small bone fragment from the proximal phalanx often occurs with this injury (Resnick, 2000; May, 2002; Greenspan, 2000) (Figure 7–17). A stress view is necessary to identify disruption of the ulnar collateral ligament of the first metacarpophalangeal joint and is usually obtained whenever there is a question of injury to this joint (Bohndorf and Kilcoyne, 2002). MRI is also an imaging option for investigation of this injury.

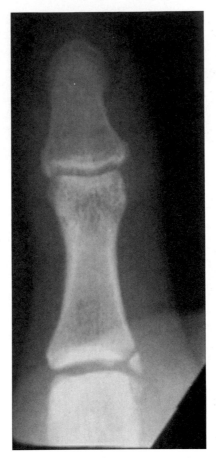

Figure 7–17 A small avulsion fracture at the base of the proximal first phalanx. Such a lesion some-times accompanies a rupture of the ulnar collateral ligament of the first metacarpophalangeal joint.

Dislocations and instability are common pathologies among the carpal bones and tend to occur in predictable patterns. Disruption of the radioscaphoid and scapholunate ligaments results in scapholunate dissociation. Widening of the space between the scaphoid and lunate on a posterior to anterior radiograph is apparent with this ligamentous injury, particularly when the fist is clenched (Resnick, 2000) (Figure 7–18). Scapholunate ligament injury may be suspected with widening of the scapholunate interval of greater than 2 mm on the PA radiograph. A gap of 4 mm is considered pathognomonic. Another common plain film finding of scapholunate dissociation is the so-called cortical ring sign or signet ring sign. These descriptions refer to abnormal orientation of the scaphoid resulting in the carpal being volarly rotated and appearing foreshortened on the PA radiograph. Rather than the usual trapezoidal appearance, the change in tilt now results in a triangular shape (Greenspan, 2000; Resnick, 2000; May, 2000).

Fractures of the shaft of the phalanges are also relatively common and easily recognized, but displacement and angulation are a concern for outcomes (Resnick, 2000).

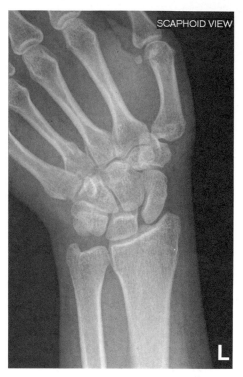

Figure 7–18 A PA view of the wrist reveals increased space between the scaphoid and lunate suggesting disruption of the interposed ligaments.

Dislocations and fracture dislocations to the proximal interphalangeal (PIP) joints are common and may include periarticular soft tissue injury. If hyperextension is the mechanism, avulsion of the volar plate from the base of the middle phalanx often occurs and can best be viewed by a lateral view radiograph. Medial and lateral fractures may include injury to the collateral ligaments (May, 2002; Resnick, 2000) (Figure 7–19).

Injuries to the proximal margins of the distal interphalangeal (DIP) joints are also common. So-called mallet fractures or baseball fractures occur with externally forced flexion of the distal phalanx as a small fragment of the distal phalanx may be avulsed by the extensor hood. Many of these injuries do not actually involve fractures and are negative radiographically. If a bone fragment is avulsed with the distal attachment of the extensor mechanism, radiographs are usually revealing (May, 2002; Bendre et al., 2005) (Figure 7–20).

Radiographs reveal many of the characteristic tissue changes associated with rheumatoid arthritis, but may not be particularly sensitive to early erosive bone lesions or inflamed synovial tissue (Backhaus, 1999; Backhaus, 2002). Involvement of the wrist is seen in almost all patients with rheumatoid arthritis, and some of the earliest involvement is at the distal radioulnar and radiocarpal joints. Typical findings associated with rheumatoid arthritis include:

1. Soft tissue swelling from joint effusion and synovial proliferation.

2. Periarticular osteopenia early in the disease with progression to generalized form later.

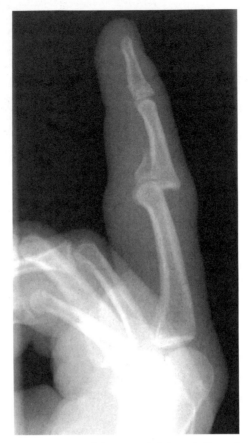

Figure 7–19 A lateral view radiograph of the second digit, revealing a fracture dislocation of the PIP joint.

3. Uniform joint space narrowing.

4. Bony erosions often occur at the distal radioulnar joint, radial and ulnar styloid processes, waist of the scaphoid, radial aspect of the second and third metacarpal heads, metacarpophalangeal and PIP joints; the DIP joints are often spared early in the disease, but may become involved later.

5. Cyst or pseudocyst formation.

In advanced rheumatoid disease, the entire carpus may translocate ulnarly and may be accompanied by other instabilities such as dissociations at the distal radioulnar and scapholunate articulations. Dorsal and volar carpal instabilities are also common as are ulnar drift, swan neck, and boutonnière deformities in the digits (El-Khoury et al., 2003a; Manaster, 2002) (Figure 7–21).

The hand is a frequent site of osteoarthritis, although some joints are affected preferentially. Osteoarthritis routinely occurs at the first carpometacarpal joint, the PIP joints, and the DIP joints. The presence of Bouchard's nodes proximally and Heberden's nodes

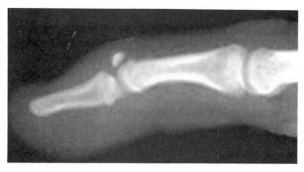

Figure 7–20 This lateral view radiograph of a digit demonstrates the small avulsion fracture of the distal phalanx typical of mallet finger.

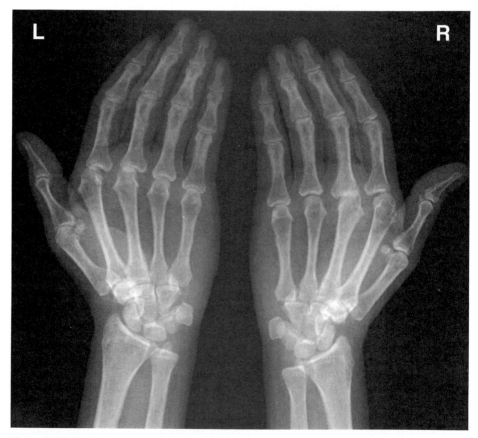

Figure 7–21 A AP view of the hands in this 59-year-old female with rheumatoid arthritis. Erosive changes are not prominent, but subluxations of the left first through third metacarpophalangeal joints and right second and third metacarpophalangeal joints are clearly evident.

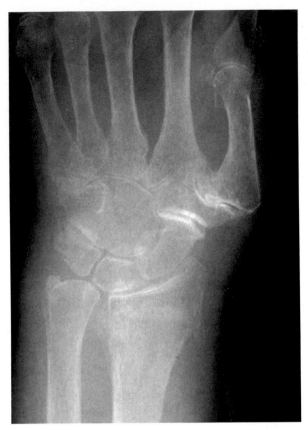

Figure 7–22 This PA view of the wrist reveals multiple findings. Accompanying the distal radius fracture in this 79-year-old female is considerable demineralization of the bones and changes consistent with degenerative joint disease. At the first carpometacarpal joint and the articulation of the scaphoid and trapezium, note the subchondral sclerosis, loss of joint space, and remodeling.

distally may offer an external indication of ongoing articular degenerative change. Another common site of involvement is the scaphoid–trapezium–trapezoid complex. Osteoarthritis of the distal radioulnar, radiocarpal, and second through fifth metacarpophalangeal joints is uncommon in the absence of trauma or an underlying disease process causing predisposition. Typical radiographic findings consistent with this diagnosis include joint space narrowing, marginal osteophyte formation, subchondral sclerosis, and subchondral cysts (Manaster, 2002; El-Khoury, 2003b; Greenspan, 2000) (Figure 7–22).

COMPUTED TOMOGRAPHY

If radiography is indefinite or fails to provide adequate detail for decision making, CT may provide further clarification. Fracture lines and fragment locations can best be delineated with the help with CT. The CT sections reconstructed at right angles to the fracture lines are particularly revealing (Goldfarb et al., 2001). Multidetector CT has been found to identify radiographically occult carpal fractures as well as rule out fractures as the cause of persistent wrist pain. When fractures are present, the images provided by multidetector CT reveal precise fracture anatomy with remarkable accuracy (Kiuru et al., 2004). Thus, the fractures delineated in the prior section, while often viewed adequately with radiography, are imaged in greater detail with CT.

Subluxation of the distal radioulnar joint is well demonstrated on CT (Greenspan, 2000; Rosner, 2004; Resnick, 2000). CT has been particularly cited as being valuable in accurately assessing hook of the hamate fractures (Greenspan, 2000; Rosner, 2004; Resnick, 2000) (Figures 7–23 and 7–24). Fracture–dislocations across the carpus are better demonstrated on CT than in radiography (Kaneko et al., 2002; Garavaglia et al., 2004). Similarly, triquetral fractures, which may include avulsion injuries are better visualized with CT (Goldfarb et al., 2001).

Accurate assessment of the reorientation of the distal radius articular surface following fracture is critical in determining whether closed or open reduction is the preferred course of action. CT has been found to allow more exact determination of the position and angle of the distal fragment for greater decision making precision, which ultimately affects functional outcomes (Cole, 1997; Rozental, 2001) (Figure 7–25).

CT may also serve a valuable role after initial diagnosis. Studies have used CT to monitor fracture healing, particularly in complex injuries (Slade and Jaskwhich, 2001; Singh et al., 2005; Plancher, 2000). For providing accurate information for clinical decision making pertaining issues such as possible nonunion and avascular necrosis, CT images in multiple planes provide bony detail greater than radiography (Figure 7–26).

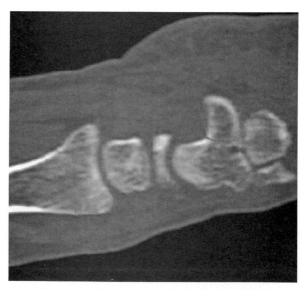

Figure 7–23 This sagittal plane reconstruction CT image through the wrist reveals a subtle fracture line through the base of the hook of the hamate.

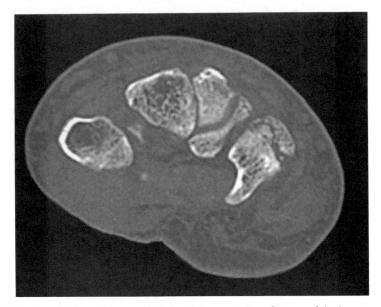

Figure 7–24 This axial view CT image of the wrist demonstrates a fracture of the hamate.

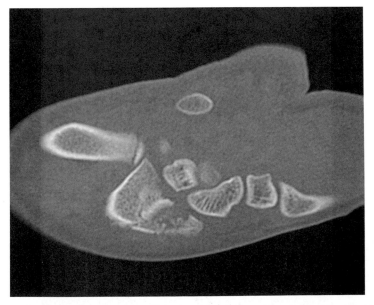

Figure 7–25 The oblique reconstruction CT image through the wrist reveals a comminuted fracture of the distal radius.

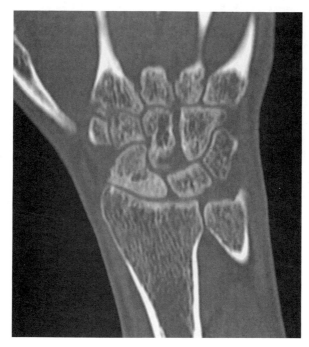

Figure 7–26 In this coronal reconstruction, the CT image reveals sclerosis of the proximal portion of the scaphoid, which is consistent with developing avascular necrosis.

Tumors of the hand and wrist most frequently develop from dystrophic lesions while neoplastic disease is rare. Because of multiplanar capability and excellent tissue contrast, MRI and CT are used in the assessment of suspicious masses, although CT is still the method of choice in assessing small bone tumors such as osteoid osteoma (Garcia and Bianchi, 2001).

 MAGNETIC RESONANCE IMAGING

Although CT is valuable in assessing the stability of the distal radioulnar joint, MRI offers the advantage of concurrently imaging the neighboring soft tissues. MRI allows direct visualization of the dorsal and volar radioulnar ligaments, allowing assessment of their integrity (Rosner et al., 2004; Steinbach and Smith, 2000). Injury to the TFCC can occur as a result of trauma or as sequela from instability at the distal radioulnar joint or from a past fracture of the distal radius (resulting in shortening) (Greenspan, 2000; Rosner et al., 2004). Pain and tenderness along the ulnar aspect of the wrist, which are irritated by wrist and forearm motion, are common (Rosner et al., 2004). The disk normally appears as a biconcave structure of low signal intensity on T1-weighted images (Greenspan, 2000). The value of MRI in detecting TFCC pathology is limited owing to similar findings on images of asymptomatic subjects, particularly with advancing age (Rosner et al., 2004; Bohndorf and Kilcoyne, 2002; May, 2002; Morley, 2001; Kato et al., 2000). Thus, the findings consistent with injury warrant cautious interpretation. Injury can occur to the disk or the ligamentous attachments (Rosner et al., 2004; May, 2002). Traumatic injuries tend to occur at the radial attachment, whereas degenerative tears tend to occur centrally where the disk is thin (Rosner et al., 2004; Farooki et al., 2003). Tears appear as increased signal intensity on T2-weighted images, demonstrating continuity between the normally separate radiocarpal and distal radioulnar joints (Farooki et al., 2003; Greenspan, 2000). Partial tears demonstrate high signal intensity on either side of the surface of the disk, but without continuity through the midsubstance (Farooki et al., 2003). The radial insertion of the disk contains hyaline cartilage and tends to be high signal intensity and must not be mistaken for a tear (Farooki et al., 2003). A degenerative tear demonstrates increased signal intensity centrally, where the disk is naturally thin (Rosner et al., 2004; Farooki et al., 2003). If the ligamentous attachments are torn, the altered morphology of the ligaments will usually be evident (Rosner et al., 2004). Arthrography and magnetic resonance arthrography are generally considered more accurate in demonstrating frank tears of the TFCC than conventional MRI (Elentuck and Palmer, 2004; Rosner et al., 2004; DeSmet, 2005). Arthrography or magnetic resonance arthrography allow diagnosis of tears by contrast extravasation from within the wrist to the normally anatomically separate distal radioulnar joint. This finding must also be interpreted with caution because communication of the two compartments has been found in asymptomatic as well as symptomatic persons (Steinbach and Smith, 2000; Cerezal et al., 2005; De Smet, 2005) (Figure 7–27).

Ulnar impaction or abutment syndrome is a degenerative disorder in which the distal lateral ulna compresses the TFCC and proximal medial lunate. Associated with a positive ulnar variance, MRI usually reveals subchondral sclerosis or subchondral cyst formation within the lunate or ulnar head along with tears or perforations of the triangular fibrocartilage. The lunatotriquetral ligament may also be affected (Steinbach and Smith, 2000; May, 2002) (Figure 7–28).

MRI is typically not the imaging modality of choice for detecting fracture, but the scaphoid is an exception. Prior to the advent of more sophisticated imaging modalities, repeat conventional radiography was used for possible occult fractures of the scaphoid, but is no longer supported by the literature (Low and Raby, 2005; Tiel van Buul et al., 1995). CT and scintigraphy offer greater sensitivity of fracture detection than does radiography. CT, however, relies upon cortical and trabecular displacement for signal change, which are not always present in scaphoid fractures (Groves et al., 2005; Temple, 2005). Bone scans consistently identify areas of increased mineral turnover associated with scaphoid fractures to result in greater sensitivity than conventional radiography (Fowler et al., 1998; Roolker et al., 1997; Tiel van Buul, 1995; Murphy and Eisenhauer, 1994), but scintigraphy imaging may require passage of several days after onset for accuracy (Murphy et al., 1995; Fowler et al.,1998). Recent studies have also suggested high-spatial resolution ultrasonography to be of value in detecting scaphoid fractures, but this modality is yet to be generally accepted (Hauger et al., 2002; Herneth et al., 2001). Multiple studies have supported the use of MRI for investigation of scaphoid fractures, reporting 95 to 100 percent levels of sensitivity (Moller et al., 2004; Brydie and Raby, 2003; Gaebler et al., 1998; Hunter et al., 1997; Breitenseher et al., 1997). The diagnosis of a

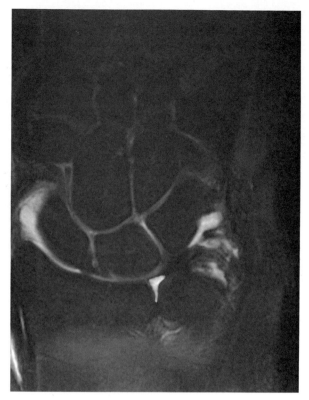

Figure 7–27 This MR image subsequent to injection of gadolinium reveals fenestration of the TFCC and a complex tear with fraying of the radiocarpal side, allowing the fluid to tract within the TFCC and proximally.

fracture of the scaphoid on MRI is made when there is evidence of a discrete low signal line which traverses the scaphoid from cortex to cortex on T1-weighted images with a corresponding area of high signal on the T2-weighted or short tau inversion recovery (STIR) images (Brydie and Raby, 2003; Farooki et al., 2003). Other investigators have used broader diagnostic criteria including the presence of any signal abnormality, be it the usually present marrow edema or a linear signal suggesting macrofracture (Brooks et al., 2005) (Figure 7–29). Correct identification of a scaphoid fracture is imperative for appropriate management because of the risk of nonunion and avascular necrosis. If scaphoid injury progression to avascular necrosis occurs, the MRI features of bone necrosis include replacement of normal fatty marrow with edema (low signal on T1-weighted images and bright on T2-weighted images) or fibrosis (dark on both sequences) (Steinbach and Smith, 2000). MRI is currently the preferred imaging modality for differential diagnosis because it allows for rapid detection and prompt determination of the optimal course of care, thereby minimizing unnecessary immobilization (Brydie and Raby, 2003) (Figure 7–30).

MRI of suspected carpal fractures following radiography has resulted in identification of false-positive and false-negative initial diagnoses. Additionally, MRI identified in these

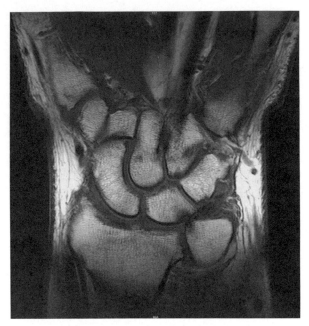

Figure 7–28 The T1-weighted MR image demonstrates the positive ulnar variance and the reactive change at the interface of the distal ulna and lunate.

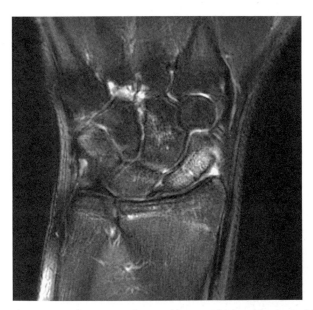

Figure 7–29 Reactive marrow changes consistent with a nondisplaced fracture of the scaphoid are evident in this T2-weighted MR image. Such nondisplaced fractures may escape detection with other imaging modalities.

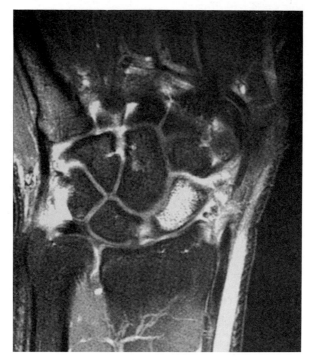

Figure 7–30 In this MR with the addition of contrast, the middle and distal portions of the scaphoid are enhanced, which is consistent with hypervascular activity after a fracture. The most proximal portion of the bone, however, does not enhance, which is consistent with early avascular necrosis.

patients' soft tissue injuries which were previously not noted. Thus, MRI results have been found to change the course of clinical management substantially with identification of previously occult fractures (Brydie and Raby, 2003; Brooks et al., 2005; Kumar et al., 2005). The high costs of MRI, however, make standard use for acute wrist lesions impractical (Mack et al., 2003).

Instability in the wrist is a frequent occurrence. The lunate is the most dislocated single carpal bone and can occur in isolation or be accompanied by neighboring ligamentous injuries. MRI demonstrates not only the positional faults associated with these instabilities, but also the altered morphology of the ligaments, albeit in somewhat limited capacity. The progression usually begins with scapholunate dissociation occurring from disruption of the scapholunate interosseous ligament and the extrinsic supporting ligaments (Greenspan, 2000; Rosner et al., 2004; May, 2002). In addition to the widened gap between the scaphoid and lunate on a PA radiograph or a coronal slice MRI, partial or complete ligament tears can be directly detected on MRI. Discontinuity of the ligaments on T2-weighted images is strongly suggestive of a complete tear (Figure 7–31). Fluid signal around the ligament and associated bone injury may also be evident or indications of underlying injury. Partial tears more frequently involve the volar ligaments and may be demonstrated by fibrosis owing to attempts to heal (Rosner et al., 2004). Rotary

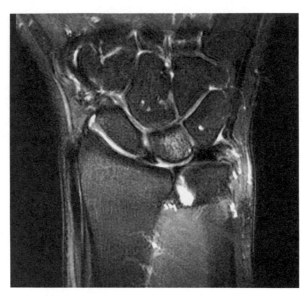

Figure 7–31 Although inconsistent to identify directly, this T2-weighted image reveals an obvious tear of the scapholunate ligament. Often, the finding is not this apparent.

subluxation of the scaphoid is also usually present (May, 2002; Rosner et al., 2004; Greenspan, 2000).

The progression of expanding instability is termed perilunate dislocation, specifically involving the capitate, due to tearing of the dorsal ligamentous attachments of the lunate (Rosner et al., 2004; Greenspan, 2000). Further progression consists of pathomechanical descriptions of dorsal and volar intercalated instability (VISI), resulting from disruption of the osseoligamentous linkages in the wrist. Dorsal intercalated instability (DISI) describes a radially oriented derangement of the wrist in which the lunate tilts dorsally and is usually accompanied by scapholunate dissociation, and a scapholunate angle of greater than 60 degrees (May, 2002; Greenspan, 2000). VISI occurs more at the ulnar aspect of the wrist and is characterized by the lunate tilting volarly, dissociation of the lunate and triquetrum from tearing of their interosseous ligament, and a scapholunate angle of less than 30 degrees (May, 2002; Greenspan, 2000; Rosner et al., 2004). Radiography often demonstrates the positional faults adequately as does MRI. MRI is only moderately consistent in allowing visualization of the ligamentous injuries as the interosseous ligaments are often not directly apparent on images (Farooki et al., 2003; Schäedel-Höepfner et al., 2001). Thus, detailed evaluation of the intercarpal ligaments may rely on arthrography, either alone or in combination with MRI (Bohndorf and Kilcoyne, 2002; Elentuck and Palmer, 2004). Computed tomographic arthrography has been suggested to be the most accurate methodology for diagnosing carpal interosseous ligament injuries (Schmid et al., 2005). The complexity of ligamentous instability in the wrist, which often accompanies fractures, exceeds the scope of this work; thus, the reader is directed to additional resources for a complete description.

As sequela to injury, the lunate is particularly susceptible to avascular necrosis (Kienböck's disease), with greater predisposition in the presence of negative ulnar variance (Steinbach and Smith, 2000; Weinberg et al., 2001). MRI is more sensitive than radiography in demonstrating early change associated with avascular necrosis. The early changes include replacement of the normal fatty marrow with edema, resulting in a low intensity on T1-weighted images and high signal on T2-weighted images. With progression, morphologic change and eventual collapse of the lunate will be evident on MRI. Degenerative change in the surrounding carpals bones may also become evident due to the altered mechanics of the wrist (Weinberg et al., 2001; Steinbach and Smith, 2000).

MRI is effective in imaging various tendinopathies of the wrist and hand. Frank ruptures of tendon, including the flexor tendons, are readily demonstrated by the loss of continuity with free edges in the low signal intensity tendons in all sequences (Steinbach and Smith, 2000; Farooki et al., 2003; Clavero et al., 2002). In general, T1-weighted images provide adequate anatomic detail for judging tendon integrity and T2-weighted images reveal hyperintense fluid signal associated with most acute pathologies (Clavero et al., 2002). Incomplete tendon ruptures or chronic tears are represented by irregular cross-sectional area, which may appear with greater intrasubstance signal intensity on T2-weighted images (Steinbach and Smith, 2000; Farooki et al., 2003). Contrast is often unnecessary, but typically shows uptake in the involved area. Postoperatively, fibrosis can be demonstrated by low signal intensity (Steinbach and Smith, 2000).

The fibro-osseous tunnels containing the flexor tendons are also susceptible to injury; their integrity or rupture is similarly demonstrated on MRI (Clavero et al., 2002; Rosner et al., 2004; Bodner et al., 1999; Martinoli et al., 2000). Injuries of the extensor mechanism are similarly visualized. Partial thickness injury to the extensor hood is represented by increased focal signal on T1-weighted images and possibly similar findings on T2-weighted images (Steinbach and Smith, 2000; Clavero et al., 2002).

The status of injuries at the insertions of tendons can also be clarified for decision making. The attachment of the extensor mechanism at the distal phalanx can be disrupted. Mallet finger or baseball finger will show a fluid signal on T2-weighted images, if not a discrete defect in continuity. Similarly, jersey or sweater finger, involving rupture of the insertion of the flexor digitorum profundus tendon on the volar aspect of the distal phalanx (classically from grasping a jersey or sweater), will reveal a similar anatomic deformity approximating the DIP joint. Retraction of the profundus tendon is common. A bone fragment avulsed from the distal phalanx may be evident in either mallet finger or jersey finger (Clavero et al., 2002; Rosner et al., 2004).

Tenosynovitis is also readily identified on MRI. De Quervain's tenosynovitis, involving the tendon sheaths of the abductor pollicis longus and extensor pollicis brevis, will be demonstrated by the inflammatory response of increased signal in the surrounding tendon sheath on T2-weighted images (Rosner et al., 2004; Steinbach and Smith, 2000; Farooki et al., 2003). Tendinosis may be represented by an enlarged tendon with increased intrasubstance signal (Rosner et al., 2004) (Figure 7–32).

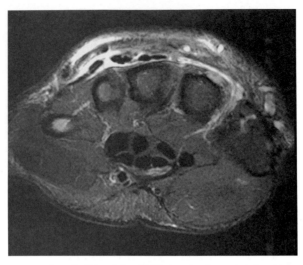

Figure 7–32 A transverse slice of a T2-weighted MRI showing increased signal intensity dorsally about the extensor tendons consistent with inflammatory response.

MRI is also accurate for examining the integrity of the stabilizing elements of the small joints of the hand, such as the collateral ligaments and volar plates. Generally, normal ligaments and tendons have low signal intensity and injury will result in increased signal intensity. Perhaps the best example of this is with injury to the ulnar collateral ligament of the first metacarpophalangeal joint or gamekeeper's thumb. Although often diagnosed from clinical examination, MRI is occasionally called upon for further investigation. MRI findings include ulnar collateral ligament disruption at the proximal phalanx base. If the rupture is frank such that the torn ligament is displaced, it often retracts to be positioned superficial to the adductor aponeurosis and is termed Stener's lesion. The retracted portion appears as a rounded or stump-like low signal structure on all sequences. Surrounding fluid signal of increased intensity often occurs on T2-weighted images. A nondisplaced tear appears as a focus of increased signal intensity between the normal ulnar collateral ligament location and bone (Rosner et al., 2004; Clavero et al., 2002) (Figure 7–33).

Injuries to the PIP joints are common and often occur to the collateral ligaments or volar plates with resultant instability. PIP joint collateral ligament injury is evidenced by discontinuity on either sequence or fluid signal on T2-weighted images on either coronal or axial slices. Medial or lateral angulation of the joint is also suggestive of collateral ligament injury (Rosner et al., 2004; Clavero et al., 2002). The presence of small avulsion fragments is also a common image finding (May, 2002). Volar plate injury often occurs from hyperextension or rotation with longitudinal compression of the joint. While demonstrated on lateral view radiographs, MRI is more sensitive and can detect avulsion injury in the presence or absence of a displaced bone fragment. Additionally, MRI allows assessment of the surrounding soft tissue. Disruption suggests complete injury, whereas subtle injury may demonstrate increased intrasubstance signal intensity of the volar plate (May, 2002; Clavero et al., 2002; Rosner et al., 2004) (Figure 7–34).

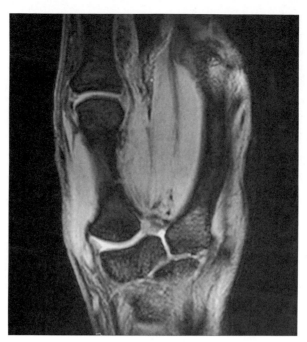

Figure 7–33 In this MR image using the Dixon fat suppression technique, a tear of the ulnar collateral ligament of the first metacarpophalangeal joint is evident. Subsequently, gapping of the radial side of the joint has also occurred. Fluid within the joint is also evident.

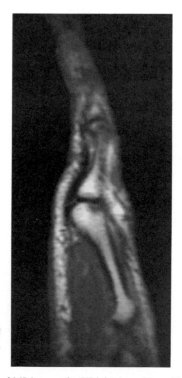

Figure 7–34 In this T1-weighted MR image, the PIP joint is positioned in hyperextension, which is consistent with injury to the volar plate.

Injuries to the central slip of the extensor tendon can be easily viewed by MRI, especially when acute clinical examination may be equivocal. Axial and sagittal images can demonstrate tears of the central slip by virtue of tendon fiber disruption being evident (Clavero et al., 2002). These injuries may evolve into boutonnière deformities with flexion of the proximal joint and extension of the distal joint. Such deformities may occur from trauma, but also as part of the spectrum of tissue changes in the hands and wrists from rheumatoid or another inflammatory arthritis (Greenspan, 2000; May, 2002; Rosner, 2004) (Figures 7–35 and 7–36). Other common findings for which MRI has greater sensitivity than radiography, particularly early in the course of the disease include (Ostergaard and Szkudlarek, 2001; Peterfy, 2001; Backhaus et al., 1999; Backhaus et al., 2002):

1. Synovitis is usually demonstrated with thicker than normal synovium in articular and peritendinous structures, which is further delineated with marked enhancement after administration of gadolinium.

2. Bone erosion is typically evident within well-defined margins as areas of decreased intensity of low signal cortical bone and loss of high signal trabecular bone.

3. Bone marrow edema is depicted by increased signal intensity on T2-weighted images and decreased signal on T1-weighted images within trabecular bone.

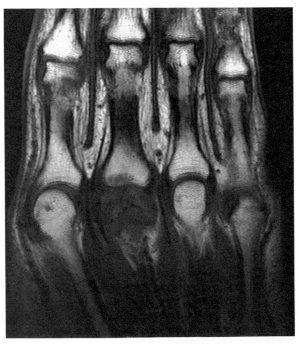

Figure 7–35 In this T1-weighted MR image of the metacarpophalangeal joints of a woman with rheumatoid arthritis, erosive destruction of the head of the second metacarpal joint is present.

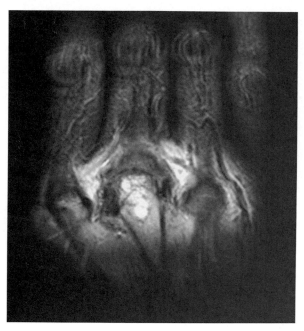

Figure 7–36 In the T2-weighted MR image of the same patient as in Figure 7–35, the increased signal intensity enveloping the second metacarpophalangeal joint is consistent with extensive synovitis.

ULTRASOUND

Ultrasound has long been considered an attractive option for imaging soft tissues owing in part to its convenience and modest cost. Image quality, however, has historically not been consistent with desired levels of clinical accuracy. Recent technologic advances with high-resolution transducers and signal processing has allowed for remarkable changes in image quality and growing acceptance in clinical application (Middleton et al., 2001).

Ultrasound has been found to be very sensitive in detection of synovitis and tenosynovitis, typical of rheumatoid arthritis (Figure 7–37). Sensitivity to erosive lesions of bone, however, is less than desired (Backhaus et al., 1999; Backhaus et al., 2002). Lesions of the tendons, annular pulleys, and ligaments are reliably detected with ultrasound (Bianchi et al., 1999; Adler and Finzel, 2005; Lee et al., 2000). Normal tendons appear as dense linear structures readily visible owing to their relatively high level of reflectivity. With intrasubstance tearing, the parallel architecture is disturbed with less echogenicity resulting (Lee et al., 2000; Adler and Finzel, 2005) (Figure 7–38). Levels of sensitivity have been reported comparable to that of MRI in detecting annular pulley lesions (Bodner et al., 1999; Martinoli et al., 2000; Bianchi et al., 1999). Also noteworthy are reports of ultrasound offering remarkable ability to detect scaphoid fractures with investigators suggesting the possibility of high-spatial resolution ultrasound becoming an alternative to CT and MRI in detecting scaphoid fractures (Hauger et al., 2002; Herneth et al., 2001).

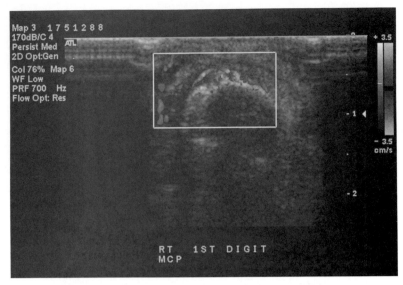

Figure 7–37 A color Doppler image suggesting thickening of the joint capsule with synovial proliferation at the first metacarpophalangeal joint. (Also see color insert).

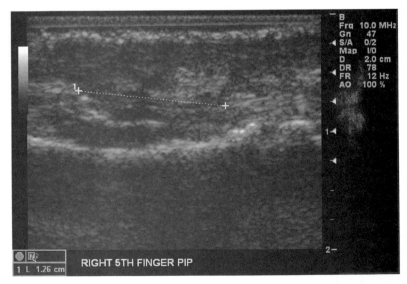

Figure 7–38 This ultrasound image is consistent with rupture of the fifth digit and is consistent with a flexor tendon rupture. Note the altered signal as measured by the sonographer across the gap of tendon retraction. *Image courtesy of Travis Fromwiller, MD, Department of Radiology, Medical College of Wisconsin, Milwaukee, Wisconsin.*

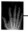 ## CLINICAL RELEVANCE TO PHYSICAL THERAPY

Rehabilitation Implications

Clinicians routinely encounter patients with hand and wrist injuries after trauma. Occasionally, the index of suspicion for unidentified injury is elevated with persistent wrist pain, particularly along the radial aspect of the wrist. Radiography is typically adequate to identify fractures of the distal radius and ulna as well as the carpals, metacarpals, and phalanges. More sophisticated imaging modalities are sometimes required to identify scaphoid fractures which have propensity for escaping initial detection. While scintigraphy and CT can contribute to differential diagnosis, MRI best identifies scaphoid fractures not initially identified by radiography. The cost of MRI and the adequacy of radiography in the majority of cases, however, do not call for routine use of MRI for all hand and wrist trauma. The cautious physical therapist will consider what imaging modalities have been used and will closely observe patients with persisting symptoms disproportionate to their known clinical picture. Patients with persistent radial wrist pain and tenderness in the anatomical snuffbox or radial aspect of the wrist may require additional imaging evaluation for the possibility of a scaphoid fracture. Identification of such an injury is of importance due to the natural history of many nonunion injuries of the scaphoid progressing to avascular necrosis and permanent loss of function.

 ## ADDITIONAL READING

Connell, D. A., Pike, J., Koulouris, G., et al. (2004). MR imaging of thumb carpometacarpal joint ligament injuries. *Journal of Hand Surgery (British), 29,* 46–54.

Cooney, W. P., Linscheid, R. I, & Dobyns, J. H. (1996). Fractures and distortions of the wrist. In Rockwood, C. A. (ed.). *Fractures in adults.* 4th ed. Philadelphia: Lippincott Raven, pp. 755–767.

Corvetta, A., Giovagnoni, A., Baldelli, S., et al. (1992). MR imaging of rheumatoid hand lesions: comparison with conventional radiology in 31 patients. *Clinical Experimental Rheumatology, 10,* 217–222.

Hashizume, H., Asahara, H., Nishida, K., et al. (1996). Histopathology of Kienbock's disease: correlation with magnetic resonance and other imaging techniques. *Journal of Hand Surgery (British), 21,* 89–93.

Imaeda, T., Nakamura, R., Miura, T., & Makino, N. (1992). Magnetic resonance imaging in Kienbock's disease. *Journal of Hand Surgery (British), 17,* 12–19.

Mikic, Z. D. (1978). Age changes in the triangular fibrocartilage of the wrist joint. *Journal of Anatomy, 126,* 367.

Owen, RA., Melton, LJ., III, Johnson, KA., et al. (1982). Incidence of Colles' fracture in a North American community. *American Journal of Public Health, 72,* 605–607.

Palmer, A. K., & Werner, F. W. (1981). The triangular fibrocartilage complex of the wrist anatomy and function. *Journal of Hand Surgery (American), 6,* 153–162.

Potter, H.G., Asnis-Ernberg, L.,Weiland, A. J., et al. (1997). The utility of high-resolution magnetic resonance imaging in the evaluation of the triangular fibrocartilage complex of the wrist. *Journal of Bone and Joint Surgery (American), 79,* 1675–1684.

Schweitzer, M. E, Brahme, S. K., Hodler J., et al. (1992). Chronic wrist pain: spin echo and short tau inversion recovery MR imaging and conventional and MR arthrography. *Radiology, 182,* 205.

Smith, D. K. (1993). Volar carpal ligaments of the wrist: normal appearance on multiplanar reconstructions of three-dimensional fourier transform MR imaging. *American Journal of Roentgenology, 161,* 353–357.

Sunagawa, T., Ochi, M., Ishida, O, et al. (2003). Three-dimensional CT imaging of flexor tendon ruptures in the hand and wrist. *Journal of Computer Assisted Tomography, 27,* 69–174.

Sunagawa, T., Ishida, O, Ishiburo, M., et al. (2005). Three-dimensional computed tomography imaging its applicability in the evaluation of extensor tendons in the hand and wrist. *Journal of Computer Assisted Tomography, 29,* 94–98.

Tomaino, M., & Elfar, J. (2005). Ulnar impaction syndrome. *Hand Clinics, 21,* 567–575.

Totterman, S., & Seo, G. S. (2001). MRI findings of scapholunate instabilities in coronal images: a short communication. *Seminars in Musculoskeletal Radiology, 5,* 251–256.

Zlatkin, M. B., Chao, P. C., Osterman, A. L., et al. (1989). Chronic wrist pain: evaluation with high-resolution MR imaging. *Radiology, 173,* 723.

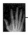 REFERENCES

Adler, R., & Finzel, K. (2005). The complementary roles of MR imaging and ultrasound of tendons. *Radiologic Clinics of North America*, 43, 771–807.

Backhaus, M., Kamradt, T., Sandrock, D., et al. (1999). Arthritis of the finger joints: a comprehensive approach comparing conventional radiography, scintigraphy, ultrasound, and contrast-enhanced magnetic resonance imaging. *Arthritis & Rheumatism, 42,* 1232–1245.

Backhaus, M., Burmester, GR., Sandrock, D., et al. (2002). Prospective two year follow up study comparing novel and conventional imaging procedures in patients with arthritic finger joints. *Annals of the Rheumatic Diseases, 61,* 895–904.

Bendre, A., Hartigan, B., & Kalainov, D. (2005). Mallet finger. *Journal of the American Academy of Orthopedic Surgery, 13,* 336–44.

Bianchi, S., Martinoli, C., & Abdelwahab, I. F. (1999). High-frequency ultrasound examination of the wrist and hand. *Skeletal Radiology*, 28, 121–129.

Bodner, G., Rudisch, A., Gabl, M., et al. (1999). Diagnosis of digital flexor tendon pulley disruption: a comparison of high frequency ultrasound and MRI. *Ultraschall in der Medizin, 20,* 131–136.

Bohndorf, K., & Kilcoyne, R. F. (2002). Traumatic injuries: imaging of peripheral musculoskeletal injuries. *European Radiology, 12,* 1605–1616.

Brandser, EA., & Ellington, B. T. (2000). Macho fracture: distal fifth metacarpal fracture revisited. *Emergency Radiology, 7,* 349–351.

Breitenseher, M. J., Metz, V. M., Gilula, L. A., et al. (1997). Radiographically occult scaphoid fractures: value of MR imaging in detection. *Radiology, 203,* 245–250.

Brondum, V., & Larsen, C. (1992). Fracture of the carpal scaphoid: frequency and distribution in a well defined population. *European Journal of Radiology, 15,* 118–122.

Brooks, S., Cicuttini, F., Lim, S., et al. (2005). Cost effectiveness of adding magnetic resonance imaging to the usual management of suspected scaphoid fractures. *British Journal of Sports Medicine, 39,* 75–79.

Brydie, A., & Raby, N. (2003). Early MRI in the management of clinical scaphoid fracture. *British Journal of Radiology, 76,* 296–300.

Cerezal, L., Abascal, F., Garcia-Valtuille, R., & Del Pinal R. (2005). Wrist MR arthrography: how, why, when. *Radiologic Clinics of North America, 43,* 43:709–731.

Clavero, JA., Alomar, X, Monill, JM., et al. (2002). MR imaging of ligament and tendon injuries of the fingers. *Radiographics, 22,* 237–256.

Cole, R., Bindra, RR., Evanoff, BA., et al. (1997). Radiographic evaluation of osseous displacement following intra-articular fractures of the distal radius: reliability of plain radiography versus computed tomography. *Journal of Hand Surgery (American), 22,* 792–800.

Colles, A. (1972). The classic: on the fracture of the carpal extremity of the radius (reprinted from original 1814 article). *Clinical Orthopaedics and Related Research, 83,* 3–5 (abst.).

De Smet, L. (2005). Magnetic resonance imaging for diagnosing lesions of the triangular fibrocartilage complex. *Acta Orthopaedica Belgica, 71,* 396–398.

Elentuck, D., & Palmer, W. (2004). Direct magnetic resonance arthrography. *European Radiology, 14,* 1956–1967.

El-Khoury, G., Stanley, M., & Bennett, D. (2003a). Rheumatoid arthritis. In: El-Khoury, G. (ed.). *Essentials of Musculoskeletal Imaging.* Philadelphia: Churchill Livingstone.

El-Khoury, G., Stanley, M., & Bennett, D. (2003b). Rheumatoid arthritis. In: El-Khoury, G: (ed.). *Essentials of Musculoskeletal Imaging.* Philadelphia: Churchill Livingstone.

Farooki, S., Ashman, C., & Yu, J. (2003). Wrist. In: El Khoury, G. (ed.). *Essentials of musculoskeletal imaging.* Philadelphia: Churchill Livingstone.

Fowler, C., Sullivan, B., Williams, L., et al. (1998). A comparison of bone scintigraphy and MRI in the early diagnosis of the occult scaphoid waist fracture. *Skeletal Radiology, 27,* 683–687.

Gaebler, C., Kukla, C., Breitenseher, M., et al. (1996). Magnetic resonance imaging of occult scaphoid fractures. *Journal of Trauma, 41,* 73–76.

Garcia, J., & Bianchi, S. (2001). Diagnostic imaging of tumors of the hand and wrist. *European Radiology, 11,* 1470–1482.

Garavaglia, G., Bianchi, S., Santa, D., & Fusetti, C. (2004). Trans-trapezium carpometacarpal dislocation of the thumb. *Archives of Orthopaedic and Trauma Surgery, 124,* 67–68.

Goldfarb, C. A., Yin, Y, Gilula, L. A., et al. (2001). Wrist fractures: what the clinician wants to know. *Radiology, 219,* 11–28.

Greenspan, A. (2000). *Orthopedic radiology.* 3rd ed. Philadelphia : Lippincott Williams & Wilkins.

Groves, A., Cheow, H., Balan, K., et al. (2005). Case report: false negative 16 detector multislice CT for scaphoid fracture. *British Journal of Radiology, 78,* 57–79.

Hauger, O, Bonnefoy, O, Moinard, M., et al. (2002). Occult fractures of the the waist of the scaphoid: early diagnosis by high-spatial resolution sonography. *American Journal of Roentgenology, 178,* 1239–1245.

Herneth, A., Siegmeth, A., Bader, T., et al. (2001). Scaphoid fractures: evaluation with high-spatial resolution US initial results. *Radiology, 220,* 231–235.

Hunter, J., Escobedo, E, Wilson, A., et al. (1997). MR imaging of clinically suspected scaphoid fractures. *American Journal of Roentgenology, 1168,* 287–293.

Jeong, G., Kram, D., & Lester, B. (2001). Isolated fracture of the trapezoid. *American Journal of Orthopedics, 30,* 228–230.

Kaneko, K., Ono, A., Uta, S., et al. (2002). Hamatometacarpal fracture dislocation: distinctive three dimensional computed tomographic appearance. *Chirugie de la Main, 21,* 41–45.

Kato, H., Nakamura, R., Shionoya, K., et al. (2000). Does high-resolution MR imaging have better accuracy than standard MR imaging for evaluation of the triangular fibrocartilage complex? *Journal of Hand Surgery (British), 25,* 487–491.

Kiuru, M. J., Haapamaki, V. V, Koivikko, M. P., & Koskinen, S. K. (2004). Wrist injuries: diagnosis with multidetector CT. *Emergency Radiology, 10,* 182–185.

Kumar, S., O'Connor, A., Despois, M., & Galloway, H. (2005). Use of early magnetic resonance imaging in the diagnosis of occult scaphoid fractures: the CAST study. *New Zealand Medical Journal, 118,* U1296.

Lee, D., Robbin, M., Galliott, R., & Graveman, V. (2000). Ultrasound evaluation of flexor tendon lacerations. *Journal of Hand Surgery (American), 25,* 236–241.

Leslie, I. J., & Dickson, R. A. (1981). The fractured carpal scaphoid. Natural history and factors influencing outcome. *Journal of Bone and Joint Surgery (British), 63,* 225–230.

Low, G., & Raby, N. (2005). Can follow-up radiography for acute scaphoid fracture still be considered a valid investigation? *Clinical Radiology, 60,* 1106–1110.

Martin, G. Mack, MG., Keim, S., et al. (2003). Clinical impact of MRI in acute wrist fractures. *European Radiology, 13,* 612–617.

Martinoli, C., Bianchi, S., Nebiolo, M., et al. (2000). Sonographic evaluation of digital annular pulleys. *Skeletal Radiology, 29,* 387–391.

May, D. A. (2002). Trauma: upper extremity. In: Manaster, B. J., Disler, D. G., & May, D. A. (eds.). *Musculoskeletal imaging. The requisites.* 2nd ed. St. Louis: Mosby.

Middleton, W., Teefey, S., & Boyer, M. (2001). Hand and wrist sonography. *Ultrasound Quarterly, 17,* 21–36.

Moller, J., Larsen, L., Bovin, J., et al. (2004). MRI diagnosis of fracture of the scaphoid bone: impact of a new practice where the images are read by radiographers. *Academy of Radiology, 11,* 724–728.

Morley, J., Bidwell, J., & Bransby-Zachary, M. (2001). A comparison of the findings of wrist arthroscopy and magnetic resonance imaging in the investigation of wrist pain. *Journal of Hand Surgery (British), 26,* 544–546.

Murphy, D., Eisenhauer, M., Powe, J., & Pavlofsky, W. (1995). Can a day 4 bone scan accurately determine the presence or absence of scaphoid fracture? *Annals of Emergency Medicine, 26,* 434–438.

Murphy, D., & Eisenhauer, M. (1994). The utility of a bone scan in the diagnosis of clinical scaphoid fracture. *Journal of Emergency Medicine, 12,* 709–712.

Ostergaard, M., Gideon, P., Sorensen, K., et al. (1995). Scoring of synovial membrane hypertrophy and bone erosions by MR imaging in clinically active and inactive rheumatoid arthritis of the wrist. *Scandinavian Journal of Rheumatology, 24,* 212–218.

Østergaard, M., & Szkudlarek, M. (2001). Magnetic resonance imaging of soft tissue changes in rheumatoid arthritis wrist joints. *Seminars in Musculoskeletal Radiology, 5,* 257–274.

Peterfy, C. G. (2001). Magnetic resonance imaging of the wrist in rheumatoid arthritis. *Seminars in Musculoskeletal Radiology, 5,* 275–288.

Plancher, K. D. (2000). Methods of imaging the scaphoid. *Hand Clinics, 17,* 703–721.

Resnick, C. S. (2000). Wrist and hand injuries. *Seminars in Musculoskeletal Radiology, 4,* 193–204.

Roolker, W., Tiel van Buul, M., Broekhuizen, A., et al. (1997). Improved wrist fracture localization with digital overlay of bone scintigrams and radiographs. *Journal of Nuclear Medicine, 38,* 1600–1603.

Rosner, J., Zlatkin, M., Clifford, P., et al. (2004). Imaging of athletic wrist and hand injuries. *Seminars in Musculoskeletal Radiology, 8,* 57–79.

Rozental, T., Bozentka, D., Katz, M., et al. (2001). Evaluation of the sigmoid notch with computed tomography following intra-articular distal radius fracture. *Journal of Hand Surergy (American), 26,* 244–251.

Schäedel-Höepfner, M., Iwinska-Zelder, J., Braus T., et al. (2001). MRI versus arthroscopy in the diagnosis of scapholunate ligament injury. *Journal of Hand Surgery (British), 26,* 17–21.

Schädel-Höpfner, M., Junge, A., & Böhringer G. (2005). Scapholunate ligament injury occurring with scaphoid fracture—a rare coincidence? *Journal of Hand Surgery (British), 30,* 137–142.

Schmid, M., Schertler, T., Pfirrmann, C., et al. (2005). Interosseous ligament tears of the wrist: comparison of multi-row CT arthrography and MR imaging. *Radiology, 237,* 1008–1013.

Singh, H., Forward, D., Davis, T., et al. (2005). Partial union of acute scaphoid fractures. *Journal of Hand Surgery (British), 30,* 440–445.

Slade, J., & Jaskwhich D. (2001). Percutaneous fixation of scaphoid fractures. *Hand Clinics, 17,* 553–574.

Steinbach, L. S., & Smith, D. K. (2000). MRI of the wrist. *Journal of Clinical Imaging, 24,* 298–322.

Temple, C., Ross, D., Bennett, J., et al. (2005). Comparison of sagittal computed tomography and plain film radiography in a scaphoid fracture model. *Journal of Hand Surgery (American), 30,* 534–542.

Tiel van Buul, M., Broekhuizen, T., van Beek, E, & Bossuyt, P. (1995). Choosing a strategy for the diagnostic management of suspected scaphoid fracture: a cost-effective analysis. *Journal of Nuclear Medicine, 36,* 45–48.

Weinberg, E. P., Hollenberg, G. M., Adams, M. J., et al. (2001). High-resolution outpatient imaging of the wrist. *Seminars in Musculoskeletal Radiology, 5,* 227–234.

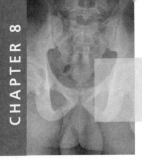

CHAPTER 8

Imaging of the Pelvis and Hip

Within the scope of this chapter, the sacrum, innominates (including the acetabulum), and proximal femur are discussed. Features of the proximal femur are of particular interest because their frequent pathologic involvement. The femoral head comprises approximately two-thirds of a sphere with an orientation medially, superiorly, and anteriorly to articulate with the acetabulum. The surface of the femoral head is covered with articular cartilage with the exception of the fovea. The cartilage is thickest centrally and is slightly attenuated peripherally; the fovea is devoid of articular cartilage. Connecting the head and the shaft of the femur is the neck extending inferolaterally. The femoral neck has considerable variability in morphology and forms an angle of approximately 130 degrees with the femoral diaphysis, which is an important angle of reference (Greenspan, 2000; DeLaMora and Gilbert, 2002). Surrounding the femoral neck are the circumflex arteries, which give rise to much of the blood supply to the femoral head. From the medial femoral circumflex artery arises the lateral epiphyseal artery, which provides the majority blood supply to the femoral head. The other important vessels are the inferior metaphyseal artery from the lateral femoral circumflex and the medial epiphyseal artery of the ligamentum teres (DeLaMora and Gilbert, 2002).

The acetabular labrum is attached at the periphery of the acetabulum and to the transverse ligament. The morphology of the labrum is triangular in the cross section and thinner along the superoanterior aspect than the posteoinferior aspect. The joint capsule connects the acetabulum to the base of the labrum and has three ligamentous condensations comprising the iliofemoral, pubofemoral, and ischiofemoral ligaments. The zona orbicularis is that portion of the capsule in which the fibers encircle the femoral neck midpoint. (Greenspan, 2000; Ashman et al., 2003).

The pelvis includes the two innominates and the sacrum, forming a strong ring-like structure. Included in this ring are the synchondrotic pubic symphysis and the two sacroiliac joints, which are a combination of synovial and syndesmotic joints. The ring-like structure is of particular functional importance as injury in one area of the ring will tend to cause disruption in another (Disler, 2002a).

 RADIOGRAPHY

Radiography remains the entry-level imaging option for many patients presenting with suspected hip or pelvic girdle pathologies, or regional manifestations of systemic disorders. After trauma, radiography is usually undertaken as the initial imaging of choice owing to the ability to obtain rapid, accurate information to guide emergent care for possible fractures or dislocations (Erb, 2001; Greenspan, 2000).

Basic landmarks guide the assessment of skeletal integrity. Shenton's line is a curve of the lower border of the superior pubic ramus and the inferior aspect of the neck of the femur, forming a smooth arc (Sanville et al., 1994; Yu et al., 2000). This arc is an important reference when considering the alignment of the femoral head and neck with the acetabulum. Ward's triangle is a radiographically lucent zone of the femoral neck located between the primary or medial compressive trabeculae, secondary or lateral compressive trabeculae, and the principal tensile group of trabeculae (Greenspan, 2000). Also in reference to the acetabulum is the identification of four fundamental osseous landmarks: iliopectineal line, ilioischial line, anterior rim of the acetabulum, and posterior rim of the acetabulum. The iliopectineal line begins at the greater sciatic notch and follows the medial cortex of the ilium and superior border of the superior pubic ramus and terminates at the symphysis. The ilioischial line begins at the greater sciatic notch along with the iliopectineal line and extends inferiorly along the ischium to the superior cortex of the inferior pubic ramus (the inferior margin of the obturator ring). The anterior rim line begins at the lateral acetabular margin and extends medially along an oblique arc that is continuous with the inferior cortex of the superior pubic ramus (the superior margin of the obturator ring). The posterior rim line begins at the lateral acetabular margin and follows a nearly straight line to the inferomedial margin of the acetabulum, just above the ischial tuberosity (Yu, 2000; Armbuster et al., 1978). Also included as a reference is the teardrop of the acetabulum, which is actually a summation of radiographic opacity due to the combined projection of the medial margin of the acetabulum and posterior acetabular wall (Disler, 2002a) (Figures 8–1 and 8–2).

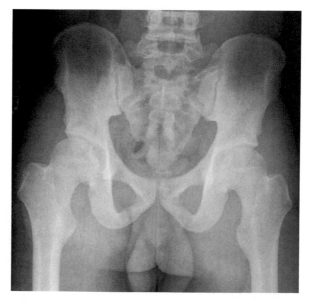

Figure 8–1 A normal-appearing AP radiograph of the pelvis in a 20-year-old male.

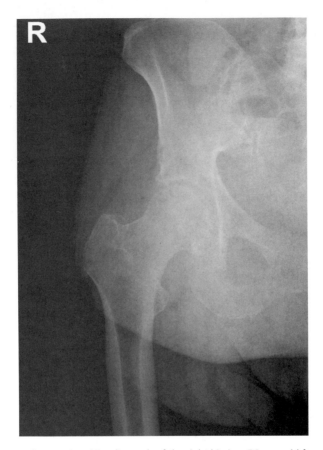

Figure 8–2 A normal-appearing AP radiograph of the right hip in a 56-year-old female.

Fractures of the proximal femur, including the head and neck, are usually diagnosed with radiographs, requiring no further workup (Greenspan, 2000; Disler, 2002a). Most hip fractures are detected with a standard anteroposterior (AP) view, but a lateral view is also required. Sites of fracture of the femoral neck are (Sanville et al., 1994; Yu, 2000; Greenspan, 2000; Disler, 2002a):

1. Subcapital–intracapsular (most common site) (Figure 8–3)
2. Transcervical–intracapsular
3. Intertrochanteric–extracapsular fracture line along the base of neck (Figure 8–4)
4. Pertrochanteric–extracapsular without and with extension into the proximal shaft as a spiral fracture

Perhaps the most commonly referenced femoral neck classification scheme is that proposed by Garden (1961, 1974).

Type I: Incomplete fracture line, externally rotated distal fragment, proximal fragment oriented in valgus, and trabeculae are parallel to femoral cortex.

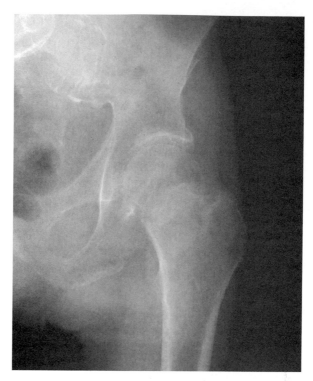

Figure 8–3 This AP radiograph from a 74-year-old male demonstrates a subcapital fracture of the proximal femur.

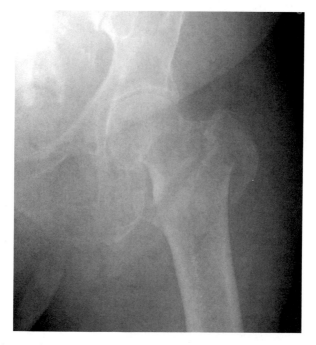

Figure 8–4 An intertrochanteric fracture is demonstrated in this AP radiograph.

Type II: Complete oblique fracture line through femoral neck, proximal fragment is undisplaced, distal fragment remains in alignment with proximal fragment, femoral head internal trabeculae are angulated approximately 160 degrees to the femoral cortex.

Type III: Complete fracture line of femoral neck with displacement of less than 50 percent, distal fragment externally rotated, proximal fragment with varus and medial rotation orientation.

Type IV: Complete fracture line through the femoral neck with greater than 50 percent displacement and dissociation, proximal fragment is relocated in acetabulum, the distal fragment is displaced proximally and is externally rotated.

Intervention for patients with proximal femur fractures will consist of open reduction internal fixation or arthroplasty (Figure 8–5). For a more thorough discussion of fracture classifications, the reader is advised to review additional orthopedic radiology resources.

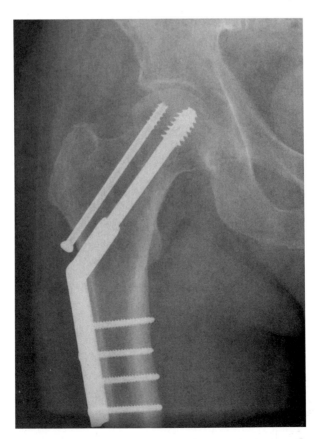

Figure 8–5 This radiograph displays an internal fixation device used subsequent to a proximal femur fracture.

Fractures of the femoral neck without displacement may, however, escape detection. Nondisplaced femoral neck or intertrochanteric fractures in the elderly may be particularly difficult to detect radiographically, but are revealed with remarkable accuracy on magnetic resonance imaging (MRI) (Verbeeten et al., 2005; Lubovsky et al., 2005; Frihagen et al., 2005; Oka and Monu, 2004).

Similarly, femoral neck stress fractures may be difficult to visualize with radiography. Initial and follow-up radiographs may be interpreted as negative. If evident, indications of fracture are likely to include a focal periosteal reaction, cortical disruption, trabecular sclerosis, and possibly new bone formation along the medial femoral neck (Ohashi et al., 1997; Erb, 2001).

If an acetabular fracture is suspected, multiple radiographic views may be required to identify all the fundamental landmarks to investigate adequately and classify the fracture, if present (Theumann et al., 2002). Classification of acetabular fractures is based on the location of the fracture and orientation of fracture lines, which are frequently determined by the position of the femoral head and the direction of force involved with the trauma. Five basic fracture patterns are typically recognized: anterior wall, anterior column, posterior wall, posterior column, and transverse (involving both columns). Wall fractures refer to the non–weight-bearing rim portions of the joints, while the column fractures refer to the weight-bearing portions of the pelvis (Disler 2002, Greenspan, 2000). Posterior column fractures are common and perhaps most important from the rehabilitationist's perspective as the fracture involves that portion of the pelvis responsible for load transmission between the spine to the lower extremity (Disler, 2002a; Greenspan, 2000). Complex fracture patterns are not unusual as fracture lines may occur in T-shaped or stellate orientations (Disler, 2002a; Greenspan, 2000). Such fractures are highly variable and difficult to categorize (Theumann et al., 2002; Yu, 2000) (Figure 8–6).

As with proximal femur fractures, pelvic fractures may escape detection if radiographic changes are subtle or patients have osteopenia or osteoporosis. Pelvic insufficiency fractures have also been reported at increased frequency in those having undergone irradiation (Ogino et al., 2003; Firat et al., 2003; Inoue et al., 2002; Huh et al., 2002).

Typical locations for pelvic insufficiency fractures include the sacrum and pubic bones along with the subcapital, intertrochanteric, and supra-acetabular regions (Otte, 1997; May et al., 1996).

Sacral fractures have become increasingly recognized as sources of low back pain in elderly patients due to osteopenia. While radiography is often the entry-level investigative technique, the fractures may escape detection. Sacral stress fractures usually parallel the sacral side of the sacroiliac joint line and are usually most detectable anteriorly (Brossman, 1999; Otte, 1997). Distinct radiographic features of stress fractures are often not visible early in the course of the disorder, but may reveal ill-defined lines of sclerosis and a focal cortical lucency surrounded by sclerotic bone formation (Disler, 2002b; Greenspan, 2000). Denis et al. (1988) proposed a classification system for sacral fractures based largely on fracture location. For more details of this classification system, the reader is referred to other radiology references.

Various classification systems for pelvic fractures have been suggested based on the apparent directional mechanism of injury, the anatomic features of the fracture, and

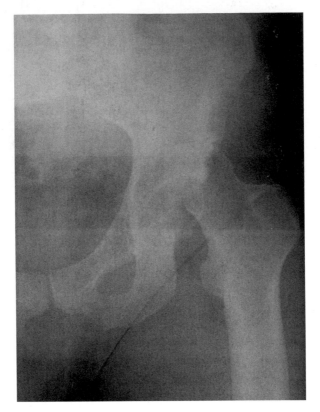

Figure 8–6 An acetabular fracture and dislocation of the hip are both evident on this AP radiograph.

whether the stability of the pelvic ring is disturbed or intact. These consider not only the bone integrity, but the function of the pelvic ring (Theumann et al., 2002; Greenspan, 2000). Perhaps the most frequently used classification by Young and Burgess takes into account description of force, direction, and severity. AP compression and lateral compression each have severity grades of I to III. Also included is a vertical shear category and combined modality to consider the confluence of more than one type of injury (Young and Resnik, 1990).

Dislocations of the femoral head can occur anteriorly, posteriorly, or centrally. Central dislocations occur as the femoral head impacts through the acetabulum from a fall onto the side of the hip, a blow to the greater trochanter, or fall from a great height. Posterior dislocation may occur from the distal femur impacting a vehicle dashboard or from a blow posteriorly onto the lumbopelvic complex while the lower extremity is stabilized in standing (Sanville et al., 1994; Yu, 2000). Hip dislocations are usually very well demonstrated on an AP pelvis radiograph, although computed tomography (CT) or MRI may be completed for consideration of loose fragments (Anderson et al., 2001). Posterior dislocation is the most common, often occurring from a force through the long axis of the femur while the hip is flexed. These are often accompanied by posterior acetabular rim fractures (Disler, 2002a; Greenspan, 2000) (Figure 8–6). Central dislocations are accompanied by acetabular fractures and are often referred to as central protrusio (Disler, 2002a; Greenspan, 2000).

Slipped capital femoral epiphysis (SCFE) occurs most commonly in young adolescents and in males more frequently than females. Rapid growth, obesity, and increased physical demand are thought to be precipitating factors. The physeal plate is obliquely oriented and susceptible to mechanical stress owing to ongoing remodeling prior to closing (Ozonoff, 1992; Reynolds, 1999; Acosta et al., 2001). Occurrence bilaterally has been reported at 20 to 50 percent, thus, suggesting the need to investigate both hips (Acosta et al., 2001; Barrios et al., 2005; Billing et al., 2004). The actual slippage is most evident with a frog-leg view because of the orientation of the slipped portion (Acosta et al., 2001) (Figure 8–7). The epiphysis is observed to slip posteromedially as the physis appears wider with less distinct margins (Disler, 2002a; Greenspan, 2000). The sensitivity rate of detection with radiography has been reported at 80 percent using both AP and frog leg views (Magnano et al., 1998; Umans et al., 1998).

Radiography offers substantial information in the study of bone lesions and remains a cornerstone in the differential diagnosis of skeletal tumors and tumor-like lesions owing to the ability to detect tumor morphologic hallmarks. Patterns of bone destruction, calcifications, ossifications, margins, and periosteal reactive changes of host bone along with specificity of location contribute to possible differential diagnosis (Priolo and Cerase, 1998; Greenspan, 2000). Radiography is, however, reported as being particularly insensitive for sacral lesions (Murphey et al., 1996; Manaster and Graham, 2003). Sacral neoplasms are most often metastases from lung, breast, kidney, and prostate carcinoma (Disler and Miklic, 1999).

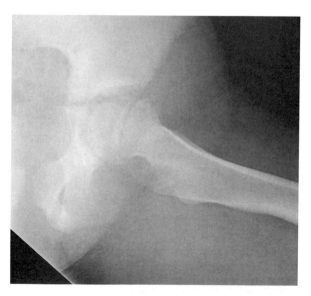

Figure 8–7 A frog-leg view radiograph demonstrating a SCFE. *Image courtesy of Travis Fromwiller, MD, Department of Radiology, Medical College of Wisconsin, Milwaukee, Wisconsin.*

Osteoid osteoma is a benign tumor which can occur in any bone, but frequently affects the proximal femur. Such lesions are most common in males in the age range of 7 to 25 years (Khoury et al., 2003). Radiographs reveal a small ovoid lucent defect with a variable degree of surrounding sclerosis and cortical thickening (Khoury et al., 2003). On MRI, marrow edema and a soft tissue mass effect may accompany (Lindner et al., 2001; Assoun et al., 1994), but may be less distinct in those having consumed anti-inflammatory medication (Khoury et al., 2003).

The manifestations of rheumatoid arthritis in the hip are typical of those found else-where and are usually evident on radiographs. These consist of (Greenspan, 2000; Murphy and Preston, 2001):

1. Osteopenia of the femoral head, particularly if steroid therapy has been utilized.

2. Loss of cartilage in a concentric pattern, although early changes may be more at the superior aspect of the joint, causing joint space narrowing.

3. Articular erosion of the ball and socket joint configuration.

4. Radiolucent synovial cysts and pseudocysts near the joint line.

5. In the advanced stage, protrusio acetabuli, where the acetabulum protrudes into the pelvis.

In assessing for the destructive changes of rheumatoid arthritis and osteoarthritis, there are two findings which tend to provide distinguishing features. The joint space narrowing with rheumatoid arthritis tends to be concentric, whereas the loss tends to be more in weight-bearing portion of the articulation with osteoarthritis (Figure 8–8) Additionally, protrusio acetabuli occurs in up to 20 percent of cases of rheumatoid arthritis of the hip, but is distinct for that disease process (Manaster, 2002a).

Radiography also usually reveals the characteristics of osteoarthritis of the hip including nonuniform superolateral joint space narrowing from cartilage loss. As the progression

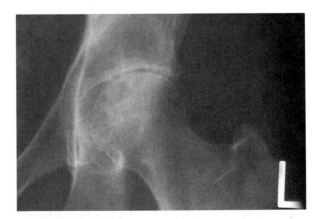

Figure 8–8 The effects of rheumatoid arthritis are evident in this AP radiograph of the hip. Erosive changes are most evident on this image. *Image courtesy of Travis Fromwiller, MD, Department of Radiology, Medical College of Wisconsin, Milwaukee, Wisconsin.*

with osteoarthritis continues; other findings include subchondral sclerosis and osteophytosis. Osteophyte formation is most frequently located at the medial femoral head and lateral acetabular rim. Additionally, new bone formation may occur along the medial aspect of the femoral neck. This finding, often referred to as bony buttressing, is almost singularly diagnostic of osteoarthritis. Another hallmark sign of osteoarthritis is subchondral cyst formation, typically at the lateral acetabulum and femoral head. Advanced osteoarthritis is characterized by remodeling of the acetabulum and femoral head (Erb, 2001; Reshnick and Niwayama, 1998; Fang and Teh, 2003; Hendrix, 2002; Manaster, 2003) (Figure 8–9).

Rehabilitation clinicians may also interact with patients having undergone hip arthroplasty (Figures 8–10 and 8–11). Critical to the long-term assessment of the integrity of hip prosthesis are comparison films completed at the time of placement. This allows visualization of possible change of position over time, which is the foremost criterion for evaluating hip prostheses components. The acetabular shell may migrate medially or superiorly, while the femoral component may rotate. Wear of the polyethylene insert is suggested by offset of the femoral head component, typically in a superior or superolateral orientation with weight-bearing (Callaghan, 2003; Manaster, 2002a). Careful examination of the bone–metal interface or bone–cement interface is in order to detect interface status on radiographs

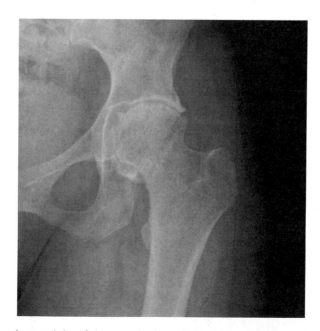

Figure 8–9 The characteristics of degenerative joint disease are well demonstrated in this AP radiograph. Note the joint space narrowing, osteophyte formation along the margins of the joint, the subchondral sclerosis of the acetabulum, and mottled appearance of the femoral head consistent with subchondral cysts.

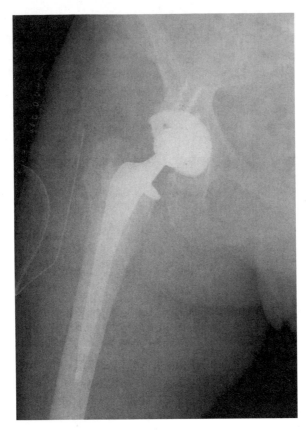

Figure 8–10 A hip prosthesis is demonstrated in this AP radiograph completed immediately post-operatively.

(Hendrix, 2002) (Figure 8–12). The criteria for assessing prosthetic components and their osseous environments are somewhat different for cemented and noncemented devices. With cemented components, small lucencies in the interface unchanging over time are considered normal. Lucencies which expand and demonstrate clear change over time suggest loosening. Cracks in the cement mantle similarly are consistent with loosening (Callaghan, 2003; Manaster, 2002a). In noncemented prosthetic components, stable fixation is represented by an absence of radiodense lines around the coated portion of the femoral portion (common around the smooth portion). Stress shielding and the spot weld phenomenon are also findings consistent with stability of the metal–bone interface. Stress shielding refers to the reduction in bone density of the surrounding proximal femur where the component has principal weight-bearing. The spot weld phenomenon is the descriptor for bone formation at the junction of the smooth and porous portions of the femoral component. An absence of these findings of stability and the presence of cortical thickening at the tip of the prosthesis or disturbance of the surface integrity of the component ("bead shedding") are consistent with loosening. Changes in lucencies are also an indicator of loosening with noncemented prostheses, but the acceptable range is less with noncemented surfaces (Callaghan, 2003; Manaster, 2002a).

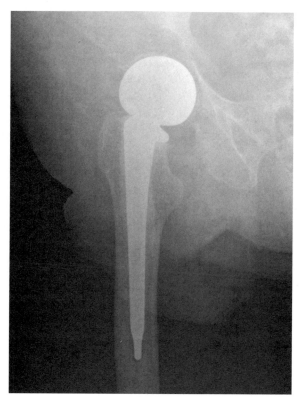

Figure 8–11 A hemi-arthroplasty of the femoral component only is demonstrated in this AP radiograph.

A recent review found that radiography offered the single highest diagnostic accuracy in evaluating aseptic loosening of the acetabular component and accuracy was enhanced by combination with bone scintigraphy (Temmerman et al., 2004). A return of ill-defined, idiopathic pain after established functional progression is of particular concern for the clinician and may be indicative of loosening of the prosthesis or other hardware complications.

Legg-Calvé-Perthes disease is an idiopathic avascular necrosis of the femoral head in children. The age of onset is typically 4 to 8 years of age when the vascular supply is most at risk. Males are much more likely to be affected. Both hips are involved 10 to 20 percent of the time, but usually not simultaneously (Manaster, 2002b; Millis and Kocher, 2003). Radiographs are usually diagnostic, but may be insensitive to early changes (Wall, 1999). The earliest radiographic changes may include effusion, arrested growth of the femoral head, and medial joint space widening. Later, fragmentation and flattening of the epiphysis occurs along with subchondral fracture. In later stages, the femoral epiphysis may return toward normal or may continue demonstrating deformity, resulting in a large, flat femoral head with a short, wide femoral neck. If the femoral head deformity continues, the acetabulum typically becomes secondarily deformed (Figure 8–13). Generally, greater age at diagnosis and female gender are risk factors for poor outcome (Manaster, 2002b; Barr and El-Khoury, 2003).

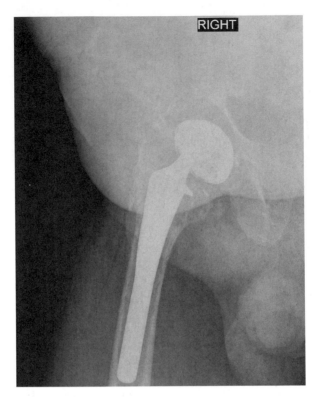

RIGHT

Figure 8–12 This AP radiograph reveals findings typical of a failing hip arthroplasty. Notice the lucency around the femoral component, suggesting space having developed at the interface of the prosthesis and bone, which is consistent with loosening. Additionally, the component positioning is suggestive of having been depressed into the femur. Further, note the femoral head component has migrated superiorly in the acetabular component.

Avulsion injuries are not common, but do occur about the hip and pelvis before skeletal maturity. Radiographs with comparison views will usually reveal the displaced fragment. Periosteum and surrounding fascia typically limit the degree of displacement (Anderson et al., 2001; Stevens et al., 1999). The exception to adequate radiographic analysis may be injury at the pubic symphysis or inferior pubic ramus as MRI may be required to detect the subchondral bone marrow change and surrounding soft tissue edema (Stevens et al., 1999). Tractional forces from musculotendinous units are usually associated with avulsion injuries. Common sites in the pelvis for such lesions include the anterior superior iliac spine (sartorius), anterior inferior iliac spine (rectus femoris), lesser tuberosity (iliopsoas), and ischial tuberosity (hamstrings), iliac crests (abdominal muscles), pubic bones (adductor muscles), and greater tuberosity (gluteal muscles) (Anderson et al., 2001; Greenspan, 2000).

Radiography also has use, albeit limited, in assessment of the pelvic girdle joints. Long-standing degenerative change in the sacroiliac joints is often evidenced by sclerosis in AP radiographs (Figure 8–14), but such findings must always be correlated to clinical signs and symptoms. Overt injury of the pubic symphysis is often readily demonstrated on radiographic AP views (Figure 8–15).

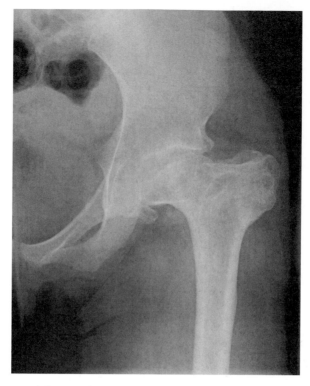

Figure 8–13 The gross deformity of the femoral head and acetabulum from advanced changes resulting from Legg-Calvé-Perthes disease as a child. *Image courtesy of Travis Fromwiller, MD, Department of Radiology, Medical College of Wisconsin, Milwaukee, Wisconsin.*

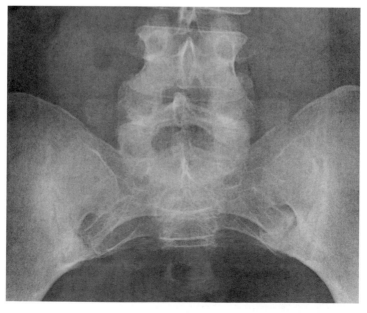

Figure 8–14 An AP radiograph demonstrating sclerosis of the sacroiliac joints in a 40-year-old female.

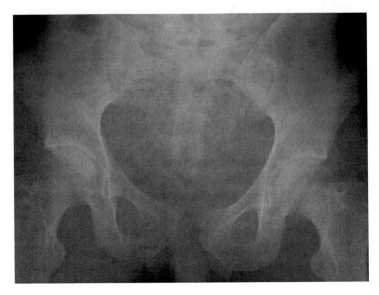

Figure 8–15 This AP radiograph in a 20-year-old male following trauma reveals diastasis of the pubic symphysis.

 ## COMPUTED TOMOGRAPHY

CT of the hip and pelvis is helpful with identifying the spatial relationships of fractures of the femoral head and acetabulum and any associated fragments. CT also has well-defined roles in consideration of congenital hip dysplasia, preoperative prosthesis planning, and neoplasms (Erb, 2001; Greenspan, 2000).

CT is frequently used to evaluate complicated fractures, particularly extending into the articular surface of the hip to assist in determining the orientation and displacement of the fracture fragments. Plain films may not be revealing because of overlying bowel gas or fracture line orientation (Hendrix, 2002; Bencardino and Palmer, 2002). In the event of trauma, CT offers the advantage of imaging for suspected pelvic fracture and to investigate for possible visceral lesions (Theumann et al., 2002) (Figure 8–16).

Insufficiency fractures of the pelvis and sacrum have been detected at 65 percent sensitivity with radiographs with a clear fracture line or osteocondensation. Bone scan has demonstrated 87.5 percent sensitivity while CT was at 98 percent (Soubrier et al., 2003).

On radiographs, sacral fractures are sometimes difficult to interpret on account of overlying soft tissues. Additionally, more evident pelvic fractures may distract the radiologist from identifying the sacral lesions. CT is of value in identifying such lesions (Diel et al., 2001). CT reveals a sclerotic band or discrete fracture lines with disruption of the anterior cortex of the sacral ala. Concurrent pelvic fractures, particularly in the pubis, are common when the origin is traumatic (Disler, 2002a; Greenspan, 2000) (Figure 8–17).

The complexity of acetabular fractures lines may present an imaging interpretation challenge, even with the addition of sophisticated options such three-dimensional and multiplane reconstruction CT. The multiplanar capabilities of CT are particularly valuable

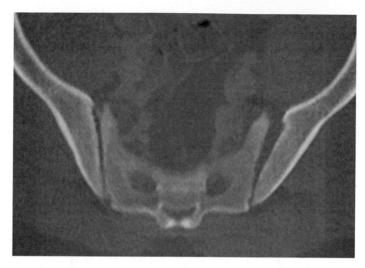

Figure 8–16 This axial CT image reveals diastasis of a sacroiliac joint subsequent to trauma.

for acetabular fractures wherein articular surface fragmentation and neighboring soft tissue injury may be inadequately represented on radiography (Figure 8–18). Fracture lines may be precisely followed and fragment locations identified, which are of great importance in preoperative planning. Additionally, CT is particularly of value in postoperative assessment of fracture alignment and healing (Greenspan, 2000; Disler, 2002a).

MAGNETIC RESONANCE IMAGING

MRI is well suited to visualize soft tissue and marrow-based abnormalities of the hip and pelvis. Owing to superb soft tissue contrast on MRI, intra-articular and extra-articular hip joint pathologies can often be readily visualized along with musculotendinous injuries. MR imaging may also be particularly of value with suspicion of occult fractures, stress fractures, and neoplasms (Figure 8–19). The capability of excellent marrow

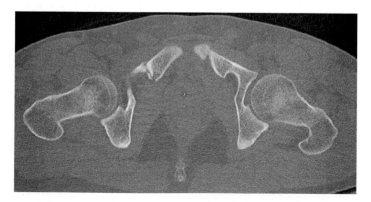

Figure 8–17 This axial CT image reveals fractures bilaterally of the superior pubic rami.

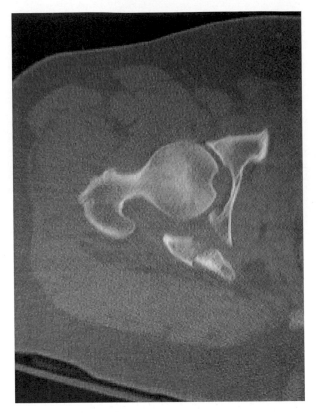

Figure 8–18 In this axial CT image, a fracture of the posterior acetabulum is demonstrated. The displacement and size of the fracture fragments are well shown by CT.

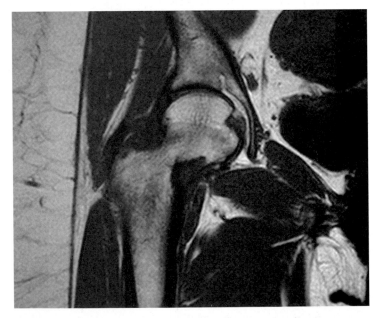

Figure 8–19 A T1-weighted MRI coronal section reveals bony change consistent with an osteoid osteoma at the neck of the femur.

contrast is specifically superior to other modalities in occult fractures (Erb, 2001; Disler, 2002b). Among the occult fractures are stress fractures, which are often classified as fatigue fractures or insufficiency fractures, depending of the preinjury status of the bone and the imposed forces. In fatigue fracture, the bone is normal, but the imposed stresses are inordinate. In insufficiency fractures, the bone strength is compromised because of underlying bone disease and is incapable of managing apparently normal loading (Overdeck and Palmer, 2004; Ashman et al., 2003).

Subchondral fractures of the femoral head, once poorly recognized, are now revealed by extensive bone marrow edema visible on MRI (Beltran et al., 2002; Bencardino and Palmer, 2002). Similarly, nondisplaced fractures of the pelvis, sacrum, and femoral neck may be particularly difficult to see with radiography. If there is strong clinical suspicion of a proximal femur fracture (such as difficulty with weight-bearing and hip pain with passive motion) in the presence of negative radiographs, further investigation with MRI is the next line of investigation (Verbeeten et al., 2005). On MRI, microtrabecular fracture is suggested by a diffuse or linear hypointense area from cortex to cortex on T1-weighted images (Figure 8–20) while increased signal intensity is evident on T2-weighted and STIR sequences, corresponding to marrow edema or hemorrhage (Bencardino and Palmer, 2002; Erb, 2001; Verbeeten et al., 2005; Lubovsky et al., 2005; Frihagen

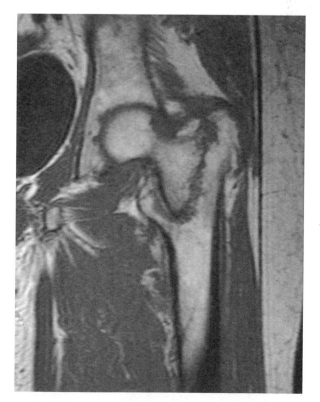

Figure 8–20 A nondisplaced fracture of the proximal femur is evident in this T1-weighted coronal section. The linear zone of decreased signal intensity spanning trochanters represents the fracture line.

et al., 2005; Oka and Monu, 2004). Prompt identification of fatigue stress fractures of the femoral neck is important owing to the potential for progression to displacement and subsequent deformity and avascular necrosis (Lee et al., 2003; Clough, 2002). The index of suspicion should always be high for femoral neck fatigue stress fractures in athletes and others engaged in activity requiring repetitive running or jumping (Clough, 2002; Overdeck and Palmer, 2004). Activity-related groin pain relieved by rest and antalgic gait are often early clinical indications of a developing fracture (Overdeck and Palmer, 2004). MRI is necessary if a fatigue stress fracture is suspected so that early identification and appropriate intervention can prevent progression to a complete fracture and the associated sequelae (Bencardino and Palmer, 2002; Clough, 2002) (Figure 8–21).

Fatigue stress fractures of the sacrum have similarly been reported in long-distance runners and military recruits with symptoms emulating disk disease. Findings on MR examination show low-signal T1-weighted images and high T2-weighted signal paralleling the sacroiliac joint. A discrete fracture line may or may not be apparent (Ahovuo et al., 2004; Major and Helms, 2000; Eller et al., 1997). Sacral insuffiency fractures are most common in the elderly and those having undergone radiation therapy (Ahovuo et al., 2004). The fractures may be radiographically occult owing to the osteopenia. With MR imaging, the fracture line is readily visible as linear low to intermediate signal on T1-weighted images (Figure 8–22) and increased signal on T2-weighted fat suppressed or short tau inversion recovery (STIR) sequences (Ahovuo et al., 2004; Overdeck and Palmer, 2004; Major and Holman, 2000).

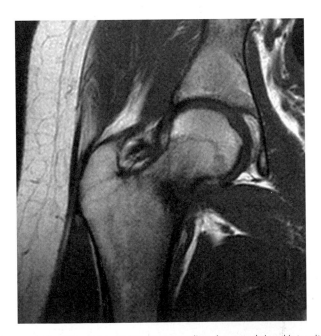

Figure 8–21 A coronal slice T1-weighted MR image revealing decreased signal intensity at the femoral neck consistent with a stress fracture in a 19-year-old female runner. Earlier radiographs were negative.

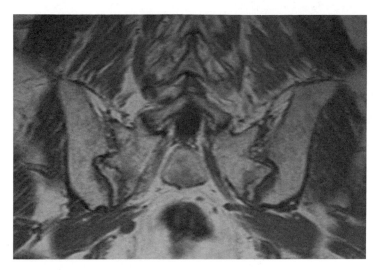

Figure 8–22 This coronal section of a T1-weighted MRI reveals insufficiency fractures bilaterally in the sacrum adjacent to the sacroiliac joints.

Radiographs investigating SCFE may be equivocal with MRI providing the necessary detail. A widened physis with increased T2-weighted signal along with displacement of the femoral head medially and posteriorly (Major and Holman, 2003) is usually confirmatory. The sagittal plane views are particularly valuable (Barr and El-Khoury, 2003). Subtle changes in the epiphyseal plate have been reported (Umans et al., 1998) visible on MRI before actual slippage and while still undetectable on radiographs. MRI has been reported to be between 88 and100 percent sensitive in identifying SCFE (Magnano et al., 1998; Umans et al., 1998).

Owing to the tenuous blood supply, avascular necrosis (or osteonecrosis) of the femoral head may result from a variety of reasons, but a frequency of 11 to 23 percent as a complication after hip fracture has been reported (Damany et al., 2005; Lu-Yao et al., 1994). Other risk factors include dislocation, SCFE, steroid use, alcoholism, and sickle cell disease (Greenspan, 2000; Manaster, 2002b). In the early stages of avascular necrosis, radiography may be normal (Coleman, 1988; Greenspan, 2000), but will demonstrate central head sclerosis if present (Manaster, 2002b). MRI is the most sensitive modality for detection of avascular necrosis, demonstrating 85 to 91 percent sensitivity (Greenspan, 2000; Manaster, 2002b). The initial MRI appearance of avascular necrosis includes somewhat nonspecific, diffuse bone marrow edema (Manaster, 2002b; Beltran, 1988). More distinct focal involvement of the femoral head later appears with a central area of fatty marrow surrounded by a serpiginous line of low signal intensity on both T1- and T2-weighted images, demarcating the peripheral aspect of the necrotic segment and a high-intensity line paralleling the low signal line on T2-weighted images. This is often referred to as the "double line sign" and is often considered pathognomonic (Manaster, 2002b; Greenspan, 2000) (Figures 8–23 and 8–24). Classification schemes for avascular necrosis have been developed and refined with the most popular by

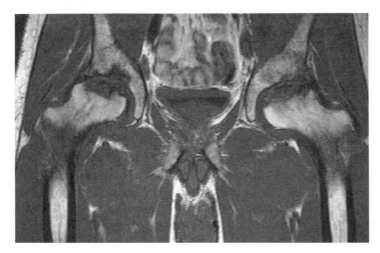

Figure 8–23 A coronal slice of the T1-weighted image reveals the destruction within the femoral heads bilaterally associated with avascular necrosis.

Steinberg (1997). Based on symptoms and image findings, this classification scheme exceeds the scope of this work; readers are referred to additional resources for greater delineation of this topic.

Appearing similar to avascular necrosis is idiopathic transient osteoporosis of the hip (TOH). This disorder has been reported with greatest frequency in young to middle-aged men and also in pregnant women (Curtiss, 1959; Guerra, 1995; Greenspan,

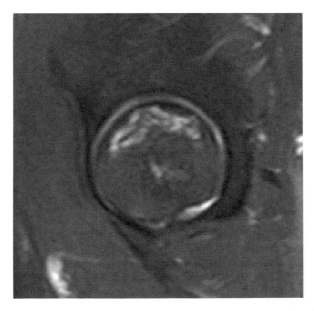

Figure 8–24 The sagittal slice of the T2-weighted image sequence demonstrates the double linear increased signal intensity characteristic of AVN.

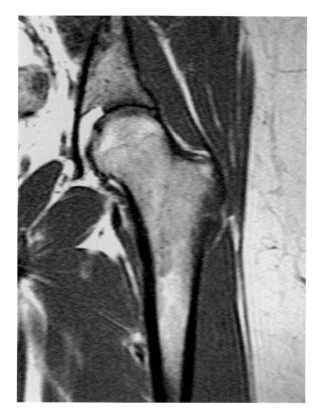

Figure 8–25 A coronal section of a T1-weighted MRI revealing decreased signal intensity consistent with transient osteoporosis in a 23-year-old female.

2000). The clinical presentation is usually one of sudden onset of severe hip pain. MRI shows low signal on T1-weighted images and high signal on T2-weighted images of the femoral head extending into the intertrochanteric region similar to avascular necrosis (Figure 8–25). Radiographs 4 to 8 weeks after onset may show osteopenia as the distinguishing factor from avascular necrosis, although precise distinction of clinical syndromes may be unclear. The natural history of the disorder is one of resolving spontaneously after several months (Disler, 2002b; Yamamoto, 1999; Hayes, 1993; Balakrishnan et al., 2003; Beltran, 2002).

The MRI appearance of the labrum is variable even in asymptomatic individuals (Cotten et al., 1998; Bencardino and Palmer, 2002; Fang and Teh, 2003). Increased intralabral signal intensities and even absent anterosuperior labra are relatively frequent findings (Cotton et al., 1998). Thus, MRI imaging has not proven highly accurate in discriminating acetabular labral pathology from the normally variable anatomy (Edwards et al., 1995; Yamamoto et al., 2005; Mintz et al., 2005). MRI may actually be more revealing of labral pathology if joint effusion is present as the joint capsule is distended, allowing better visualization of the intra-articular structures. The labrum may be outlined along with any tears (Bencardino and Palmer, 2002). Tears, when present, occur most frequently at the superior aspect of the labrum (Czerny et al., 1996; Yamamoto et al., 2004).

The most sensitive technique to image possible labral tears is MRI with intra-articular administration of gadolinium while using a smaller field of view rather than the entire pelvis (Major and Holman, 2003; Fitzgerald, 1995). The distention provided by the contrast is similar to that provided by effusion (Bencardino and Palmer, 2002). Sensitivity with the addition of gadolinium has been reported at 90 percent (Czerny et al., 1996). The most important diagnostic finding is considered to be extension of the contrast into the substance of the labrum or the interface of the labrum and articular cartilage (Plotz et al., 2001) (Figure 8–26). Correlation with clinical presentation is critical to the ultimate determination of the significance of MR arthrography findings.

Osteochondritis desiccans (OCD) and osteochondral fractures are relatively rare at the femoral head. MRI usually shows the lesions well, while radiographic findings may be subtle or normal in appearance (Beltran et al., 2002). These injuries occur most frequently in athletes and there may or may not be a history of a traumatic event. MRI often shows a wedge-shaped signal abnormality along the medial femoral head from the 10- to 11-o'clock positions. This anomaly is smaller than that present with avascular necrosis (Major and Holman, 2003). Osteochondral lesions of the hip can be visualized most frequently with T2-weighted images with possible detachment of the articular

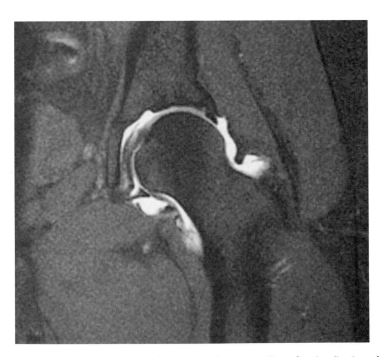

Figure 8–26 In this MR arthrogram, the distention and contrast allows for visualization of a tear of the labrum at the inferior aspect.

cartilage and subchondral bone. T1-weighted images, however, reveal the viability of bone marrow, which is an important consideration with osteonecrosis often accompanying OCD (Bencardino and Palmer, 2002).

Muscle injury can occur from externally applied force or from intrinsically generated muscle tension. Muscle strains most frequently occur approximating the musculotendinous junction. Image findings usually correlate the size and severity of the muscle injury (Smet, 1993). An acute muscle strain will usually demonstrate increased signal on T2-weighted images, reflecting the localized edema (May and Disler, 2002; Greenspan, 2000) (Figure 8–27). An acute intramuscular hematoma is likely to demonstrate increased signal on T1-weighted images because of the presence of methemoglobin, whereas an injury of longer duration is likely to have a low signal intensity rim owing to the presence of hemosiderin (May and Disler, 2002). With complete rupture, MRI allows visualization of the discontinuity of the tissue along with the hematoma. About the hip and pelvis, injury to the hamstring muscle group is frequently associated with forceful eccentric contraction (May and Disler, 2002). Tendon tears are demonstrated by partial or full-thickness fluid signal defects in the tendon with or without retraction of the torn ends (Bendcardino and Palmer, 2002). Avulsion injuries may also be investigated with MRI as the avulsed fragment is readily identifiable and increased signal intensity is seen on T2-weighted images (Brossman, 1999). On T1-weighted images, the signal may be isointense and difficult to determine as abnormal (Chung, 1999; Kingzett-Taylor, 1999).

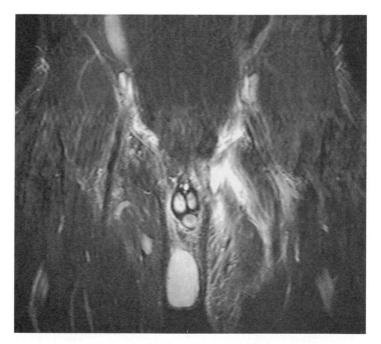

Figure 8–27 Tears of the adductor longus, magnus, and brevis tendons are evident on this STIR coronal MR image. The hyperintense signal consistent with an acute inflammatory response is typical of early-stage muscle and tendon injury.

No imaging modality has been found to identify sacroiliac joint mechanical dysfunction or offer direction as to potential treatment (Zelle et al., 2005; Lee, 2004). A number of inflammatory conditions, however, can involve the sacroiliac joint as part of a local or systemic inflammatory process. Among these are ankylosing spondylitis (AS), reactive arthritis (ReA), psoriatic arthritis (PsA), arthritis of chronic inflammatory bowel disease (AIBD), and undifferentiated spondyloarthropathy (uSpA) (Braun et al., 2000). Most common among the inflammatory conditions affecting the sacroiliac joint is AS (Zelle et al., 2005; Braun, 2000). MRI has been proven to be more sensitive than radiography in allowing recognition of the early changes within the joint. The use of gadolinium for enhancement of the joint is particularly sensitive for identifying sacroiliitis (Vinson and Major, 2003; Braun et al., 2000). Among the early changes detectable by MRI are cartilage abnormality, periarticular erosions, and bone marrow edema (Jee et al., 2004). For AS, particularly, type I lesions are patchy periarticular changes in signal intensity with low signal intensity on T1-weighted images and increased intensity on T2-weighted images (Figure 8–28). Type II lesions are low signal intensity in the subchondral bone on all sequences. Type III lesions are recognizable by a thin zone of signal intensity following that of fat along the iliac side (Yu et al., 1998; Ahlstrom et al., 1990). The most telling evidence is actual ankylosis of the joint, which can be differentiated from osteophytic bridging (Vinson and Major, 2003). For chronic changes in the joint, however, CT and radiography more readily demonstrate the bony changes than does MRI (Guglielmi et al., 2000).

Septic arthritis of the hip most frequently affects older adults and is associated with a variety of systemic or immune stressing disorders or subsequent to operative

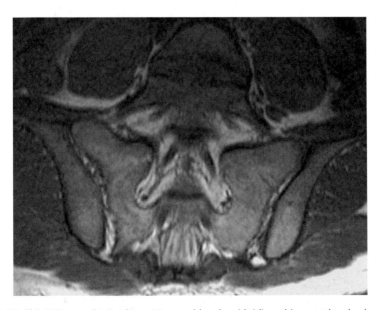

Figure 8–28 This MRI was obtained in a 19-year-old male with idiopathic onset low back pain. Note the increased signal intensity within the sacroiliac joints bilaterally consistent with sacroiliitis. The image alone is not conclusive, but raises suspicion of the possibility of very early AS and will likely be followed by additional investigation.

procedures. Early recognition and treatment is essential to a satisfactory outcome because of the rapid destructive process within the joint (El-Khoury et al., 2003; Manaster, 2002b). Suspicion of this possibility is warranted in patients who present with hip pain, antalgic gait, and fever. Early MRI findings of septic arthritis are nonspecific, often consisting of joint effusion and periarticular soft tissue edema. Cartilage loss and surface erosions are suggested as the disorder progresses (Hammond and Macnicol, 2001; Beltran et al., 2002).

Osteomyelitis of the proximal femur is represented on MRI by bone marrow edema and periostitis with soft tissue edema during the early stages followed by intraosseous abscess formation (Hammond and Macnicol, 2001). Bone marrow will have low signal intensity on T1-weighted images and increased signal intensity on T2-weighted images in acute and subacute osteomyelitis (Hendrix, 2002; Greenspan, 2000). Contrast-enhanced images (T1-weighted) are particularly sensitive in demonstrating the infectious process (Manaster, 2002b). Inflammatory arthropathies of the hip differ from osteoarthritis in the pattern of joint space loss. In osteoarthritis, the loss is predominantly superior, while arthropathies will present with more generalized loss of joint space. MRI also usually reveals effusion with synovitis and marrow edema. If infectious, areas of collection and sinus tracts may be evident (Fang and Teh, 2003) (Figures 8–29 and 8–30).

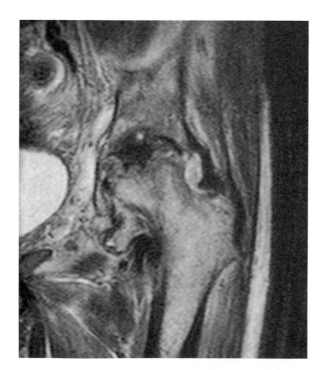

Figure 8–29 A coronal slice STIR sequence MR reveals a suspicious area of decreased signal intensity within the femoral head, possibly consistent with osteomyelitis.

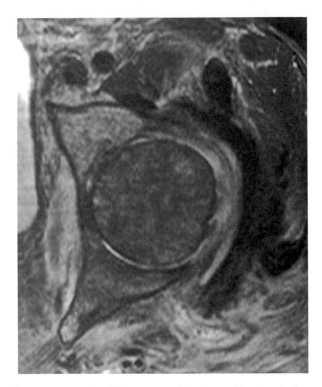

Figure 8–30 In this transverse section STIR sequence of the femoral head, note the multiple linear patterns of decreased signal intensity consistent with tract formation and characteristic of an infectious process.

Snapping hip syndrome as a general term describes multiple etiologies with a commonality of painful and audible snapping of the hip during motion. Extra-articular causes include the iliotibial band sliding abruptly over the greater trochanter and the iliopsoas over the iliopectineal eminence (Anderson et al., 2001). Such causes are usually evident on clinical examination and often do not warrant imaging. Intra-articular causes can include loose bodies, synovial osteochondromatosis, or displaced labral fragments, which are most likely to be revealed by MRI (Bencardino and Palmer, 2002; Fang and Teh, 2003). MR imaging may detect the causes of internal snapping hip syndrome (Wunderbaldinger et al., 2001), but MR arthrography is likely to be more sensitive in revealing intra-articular pathology (Disler, 2002a).

MRI is the most sensitive modality for identifying some of the features of Legg-Calvé-Perthes disease, including the early marrow edema of the femoral head. MRI, however, is often unnecessary for diagnosis as radiography is adequate. The investigational value of MRI may be important in identifying the early bony bridging across the physis later in the progression, which can result in arrest of growth (Manaster, 2002b; Barr and El-Khoury, 2003) (Figure 8–31).

MRI is also useful in differential diagnosis of trochanteric bursitis, although it is not often necessary for clinical diagnosis. In unusual cases of lateral hip pain, MRI will reveal edema in the soft tissues surrounding the bursa. T2-weighted images, especially

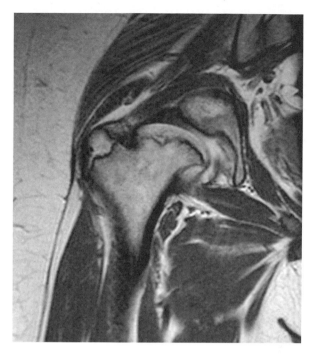

Figure 8–31 This T1-weighted image from a 14-year-old male reveals the hallmark changes associated with Legg-Calvé-Perthes disease. The femoral head is grossly flattened, particularly the epiphyseal portion, and there is widening of the femoral neck. The acetabulum is shallow and incompletely covers the femoral head.

with fat suppression, readily demonstrate the proliferation of intrabursal fluid (Ashman et al., 2003)

 SCINTIGRAPHY

Scintigraphy for the pelvis and hip is usually a secondary or complementary test. While sensitive for several disorders with the demonstration of increased isotope uptake, the level of specificity often does not allow for its use as a primary diagnostic tool (Kiuru et al., 2002). Disease of the proximal femur is a common site for pathologic fracture from metastases and the development of osteoid osteoma (Sanville et al., 1994; Greenspan, 2000). Skeletal metastases to the pelvis are relatively common because of the greater amounts of red bone marrow. Pathologic fractures are the most severe result. In asymptomatic patients, wherein a specific portion of the body cannot be targeted for further diagnostic examination, bone scanning is often used when metastases are suspected. Patients with pain or a positive bone scan are likely to undergo additional imaging such as radiography, CT, or MRI (Scutellari et al., 2000). For minimal fractures of the hip, pelvis, or proximal femur, radionuclide bone scintigraphy is sensitive, but often nonspecific, and may be negative within the first 24 hours of injury (Kwong and Sartoris, 2001).

In sacral insufficiency fractures, a linear abnormality occurs on a bone scan similar to MRI. If bilateral, the configuration forms an H, which resembles the Honda logo and is known as the Honda sign (Sundaram, 2003; Daffne, 2003).

 CLINICAL RELEVANCE TO PHYSICAL THERAPY

Rehabilitation Implications 1

Examination, diagnosis, and treatment of the pelvic girdle for mechanical pain disorders are controversial topics in the care of patients with musculoskeletal disorders. Diverse opinions exist among clinicians as to examination methodologies and diagnostic criteria for suspected pelvic girdle pain syndromes. Contributing to this controversy is the absence of a "gold standard" of diagnostic imaging, particularly for the sacroiliac joint. While MRI can demonstrate inflammatory response and bone scan indicates increased metabolic activity, these modalities offer little in assisting the physical therapist in determining a preferred course of clinical care. While radiography and CT readily demonstrate long-term change in the bone adjacent to the articular surfaces of the joint, they similarly offer little direction and such changes are common in asymptomatic persons. Thus, the value of imaging for patients with suspected mechanical disorders of the pelvic girdle is relatively limited. Exceptions to this generalization are in the presence of systemic disease or spondyloarthropathies manifest in the sacroiliac joint such as ankylosing spondylitis or other rheumatic disorders. In such cases, the imaging is not used exclusively in diagnosis, but as an adjunct procedure.

Rehabilitation Implications 2

Radiography is the first choice of physicians investigating questions of bone integrity of the proximal femur and adjacent pelvis. Because of the clear view of the structures in question and the types of pathology most frequently occurring in this area, conventional radiography is usually adequate. Two noteworthy exceptions require consideration. Extremely active or athletic individuals may present with hip pain of unknown origin and worsened by weight-bearing activity. Similarly, elderly persons may complain of idiopathic hip pain and have particular difficulty with ambulatory activity. Negative radiographs and continued clinical suspicion may warrant further diagnostic investigation. As fracture identification on radiography is typically dependent on disruption of the cortical surface of the bone, more subtle changes in bone integrity may not be readily appreciated. In both examples described above, the failure of the cancellous bone architecture may precede cortical fracture and displacement. MRI is capable of demonstrating cancellous bone edema of the neck of the femur consistent with impending failure. The clinical implications of this are quite apparent as the incomplete fracture is much more easily managed than the frank fracture and all the potential complications therein.

ADDITIONAL READING

Berg, E. E., Chebuhar, C., & Bell, R. M. (1996). Pelvic trauma imaging: a blinded comparison of computed tomography and roentgenograms. *Journal of Trauma, 41,* 994–998.

Guy, R. L., Butler-Manuel, P. A., Holder, P., & Brueton R. N. (1992). The role of 3D CT in the assessment of acetabular fractures. *British Journal of Radiology, 65,* 384–389.

Lu, Y., Fuerst, T., Hui, S., & Genant, H. (2001). Standardization of bone mineral density at femoral necK., trochanter and Ward's triangle. *Osteoporosis International, 12,* 438–444.

Peh, W. C. G., Khong, P. L., Yin, Y, et al. (1996). Imaging of pelvic insufficiency fractures. *Radiographics, 16,* 335–348.

Rogers, L. F. (1992). *Radiology of skeletal trauma.* 2nd ed. New York: Churchill Livingstone.

Sonin, A. H. (1994). Magnetic resonance imaging of the extensor mechanism. *Magnetic Resonance Imaging Clinics of North America, 2,* 401–411.

REFERENCES

Acosta, K., Vade, A., Lomasney, LM., et al. (2001). Radiologic case study. Bilateral slipped capital femoral epiphysis. *Orthopedics, 24,* 737, 808–809, 811–812.

Ahovuo, J., Kiuru, M., & Visuri T. (2004). Fatigue stress fractures of the sacrum: diagnosis with MR imaging. *European Radiology, 14,* 500–505.

Armbuster, T, Guerra, J., Resnick, D., et al. (1978). The adult hip: an anatomic study. Part 1: the bony landmarks. *Radiology, 128,* 1–10.

Ashman, C., Farooki, S., Lee, J., & Yu , J. (2003). The hip. In El-Khoury, G. (ed.). *Essentials of musculoskeletal imaging.* Philadelphia: Churchill Livingstone.

Assoun, J., Richardi, G., Railhac, J. J., et al. (1994). Osteoid osteoma: MR imaging versus CT. *Radiology, 191,* 217–23.

Anderson , K., Strickland, S., & Warren, R. (2001). Hip and groin injuries in athletes. *American Journal of Sports Medicine, 29,* 521–533.

Balakrishnan, A., Schemitsch, EH., Pearce, D., & McKee, MD. (2003). Distinguishing transient osteoporosis of the hip from avascular necrosis. *Canadian Journal of Surgery, 46,* 187–192.

Barr, L., & El-Khoury, G. (2003). Legg-Calvé-Perthes disease. In El-Khoury, G. (ed.). *Essentials of musculoskeletal imaging.* Philadelphia: Churchill Livingstone.

Bencardino, J. T., & Palmer, W. E. (2002). Imaging of hip disorders in athletes. *Radiologic Clinics of North America, 40,* 267–287.

Beltran, J., Patnana, M., Beltran, L., & Ozkarahan, G. (2002). MRI of the hip. *Applied Radiology, Nov, 33*–39.

Braun, J., Sieper, J., & Bollow, M. (2000). Imaging of sacroiliitis. *Clinical Rheumatology, 19,* 51–57.

Brossman, J., Biederer, J., & Heller, M. (1999). MR imaging of musculoskeletal trauma to the pelvis and the lower limb. *European Radiology, 9,* 183–191.

Callaghan, J. (2003). Imaging of total hip replacement from the surgeon's perspective. In El-Khoury, G. (ed.). *Essentials of musculoskeletal imaging.* Philadelphia: Churchill Livingstone.

Chung, C. B., Robertson, J. E., Cho, G., et al. (1999). Gluteus medius tendon tears and avulsive injuries in elderly women: imaging findings in six patients. *American Journal of Roentgenology, 173,* 351–353.

Clough, T. (2002). Femoral neck stress fracture: the importance of clinical suspicion and early review. *British Journal of Sports Medicine, 36,* 308–309.

Coleman, B. G., Kressel, H. Y, Dalinka, M. K., et al. (1988). Radiographically negative avascular necrosis: Detection with MR imaging. *Radiology, 168,* 525–528.

Cotten, A., Boultry, N., Demondion, X, et al. (1998). Acetabular labrum: MRI in asymptomatic volunteers. *Journal of Computer Assisted Tomography, 22,* 22:1–7.

Curtiss, P., & Kincaid ,W. (1959). Transitory demineralization of the hip in pregnancy: a report of three cases. *Journal of Bone and Joint Surgery (American), 41,* 1327–1333.

Czerny, C., Hofmann, S., Newhold, A., et al. (1996). Lesions of the acetabular labrum: accuracy of MR imaging and MR arthrography in detection and staging. *Radiology, 200,* 225–230.

Daffne, R. (2003). MRI of occult and stress fractures. *Applied Radiology, Oct,* 40–49.

Damany, D. S., Parker, M. J., & Chojnowski, A. (2005). Complications after intracapsular hip fractures in young adults. A meta-analysis of 18 published studies involving 564 fractures. *Injury, 36,* 131–141.

DeLaMora, S., & Gilbert, M. (2002). Introduction of intracapsular hip fractures: anatomy and pathologic features. *Clinical Orthopaedics and Related Research, 399,* 9–16.

Denis, F., & Davis, S. (1988). Comfort, T., Sacral fractures: an important problem—retrospective analysis of 236 cases. *Clinical Orthopaedics and Related Research, 227,* 67–81.

Disler, D. G. (2002a). Lower extremity trauma. In Manaster, B. J., Disler, D. G., & May, D. A. (eds.). *Musculoskeletal imaging. The requisites.* 2nd ed. St. Louis: Mosby.

Disler, D. G. (2002b). Metabolic bone diseases. In Manaster, B. J., Disler, D. G., & May, D. A. (eds.). *Musculoskeletal imaging. The requisites.* 2nd ed. St. Louis: Mosby.

Disler, D. G., & Miklic, D. (1999). Imaging findings in tumors of the sacrum. *American Journal of Roentgenology, 173,* 1699–1706.

Edwards, D. J., Lomas, D., & Villar R. N. (1995). Diagnosis of the painful hip by magnetic resonance imaging and arthroscopy. *Journal of Bone and Joint Surgery (British), 77,* 374–376.

El-Khoury, G., Stanley, M., & Bennett, D. (2003). Septic arthritis in adults. In El-Khoury, G. (ed.). *Essentials of musculoskeletal imaging.* Philadelphia: Churchill Livingstone.

Eller, D. J., Katz, D. S., Bergman, A. G., et al. (1997). Sacral stress fractures in long-distance runners. *Clinical Journal of Sports Medicine, 7,* 222–225.

Erb, R. E. (2001). Current concepts in imaging the adult hip. *Clinical Sports Medicine, 20,* 661–669.

Fang, C., & Teh, J. (2002). Imaging of the hip. *Imaging, 15,* 205–216.

Firat, S., Murray, K., & Erickson, B. (2003). High-dose whole abdominal and pelvic irradiation for treatment of ovarian carcinoma: long-term toxicity and outcomes. *International Journal of Radiation Oncology, Biology, Physics, 57,* 201–207.

Fitzgerald, R. (1995). Acetabular labrum tears: diagnosis and treatment. *Clinical Orthopaedics and Related Research, 311,* 60–68.

Frihagen, F., Nordsletten, L., Tariq, R., & Madsen, J. (2005). MRI diagnosis of occult hip fractures. *Acta Orthopaedica, 76,* 524–530.

Garden, R. (1961). The structure and function of the proximal end of the femur. *Journal of Bone and Joint Surgery (British), 43,* 576–589.

Garden, R. (1974). Reduction and fixation of subcapital fractures of the femur. *Orthopedic Clinics of North America, 5,* 683–712.

Greenspan, A. (2000). *Orthopedic Radiology.* 3rd ed. Philadelphia: Lippincott Williams & Wilkins.

Guerra, J. J., & Steinberg, M. E. (1995). Distinguishing transient osteoporosis from avascular necrosis of the hip. *Journal of Bone and Joint Surgery (American), 77,* 616–624.

Guglielmi, G., De Serio, A., Leone, A., & Cammisa, M. (2000). Imaging of sacroiliac joints. *Rays, 25,* 63–74.

Hayes, C. W., Conway, W. F., & Daniel, W. W. (1993). MR imaging of bone marrow edema pattern: transient osteoporosis, transient bone marrow edema syndrome, or osteonecrosis. *Radiographics, 13,* 1001–1011.

Hammond, P. J., & Macnicol, M. F. (2001). Osteomyelitis of the pelvis and proximal femur: diagnostic difficulties. *Journal of Pediatric Orthopaedics, Part B, 10,* 113–119.

Hendrix, R. W. (2002). Imaging hip and knee disorders for rehabilitation. *Physical Medicine and Rehabilitation, 16,* 539–559.

Huh, S., Kim, B., Kang, M., et al. (2002). Pelvic insufficiency fracture after pelvic irradiation in uterine cervix cancer. *Gynecologic Oncology, 86,* 264–268.

Inoue, Y, Miki, C., Ojima, E., et al. (2002). Pelvic insufficiency fractures after preoperative radiotherapy for rectal carcinoma. *International Journal of Clinical Oncology, 8,* 336–339.

Jee, W., McCauley, T, Lee, S., et al. (2004). Sacroiliitis in patients with ankylosing spondylitis: association of MR findings with disease activity. *Magnetic Resonance Imaging, 22,* 245–50.

Khoury, N., El-Khoury, G., & Bennett, D. (2003). Benign bone-forming tumors. In El-Khoury, G. (ed.). *Essentials of musculoskeletal imaging.* Philadelphia: Churchill Livingstone.

Kingzett-Taylor. A., Tirman. P. F. J., Felle, J., et al. (1999). Tendinosis and tears of gluteus medium and minimus muscles as a cause of hip pain: MR imaging findings. *American Journal of Roentgenology, 173,* 1123–1126.

Kiuru, M., Pihlajamaki, H., Hietanen, H., & Ahovuo, J. (2002). MR imaging, bone scintigraphy, and radiography in bone stress injuries of the pelvis and the lower extremity. *Acta Radiologica, 43,* 207–212.

Kwong, E. M., & Sartoris, D. J. (2001). Advanced imaging of the hip. *Applied Radiology, June,* 30–36.

Lee, C. H., Huang, G. S., Chao, K. H., et al. (2003). Surgical treatment of displaced stress fractures of the femoral neck in military recruits: a report of 42 cases. *Archives of Orthopaedic and Trauma Surgery, 123,* 527–533.

Lee, D. (2004). *The pelvic girdle.* 3rd ed. London: Churchill Livingstone.

Lindner, N. J., Ozaki, T., Roedl, R., et al. (2001). Percutaneous radiofrequency ablation in osteoid osteoma. *Journal of Bone and Joint Surgery (British), 83,* 391–396.

Lubovsky, O., Liebergall, M., Mattan, Y, et al. (2005).Early diagnosis of occult hip fractures. MRI versus CT scan. *Injury, 36,* 788–792.

Lu-Yao, G., Keller, R., Littenberg, B., & Wennberg, J. (1994). Outcomes after displaced fractures of the femoral neck: a meta-analysis of one hundred and six published reports. *Journal of Bone and Joint Surgery (American), 76,* 5–25.

Magnano, G. M., Lucigrai, G., De Filippi, C., et al. (1998). Diagnostic imaging of the early slipped capital femoral epiphysis. *Radiologica Medica (Torino), 95,* 16–20.

Major, N. M., & Helms, C. A. (2000). Sacral stress fractures in long distance runners. *American Journal of Roentgenology, 174,* 727–729.

Major, N. M., & Holman, W. R. (2003). MR imaging of the hip and pelvis: current concepts. *Applied Radiology, June,* 14–21.

Manaster, B., & Graham, T. (2003). Imaging of sacral tumors. *Neurosurgical Focus, 15,* E2.

Manaster B. (2002a). Arthritis. In Manaster, B. J., Disler, D. G., & May, D. A. (eds.). *Musculoskeletal imaging. The requisites.* 2nd ed. St. Louis: Mosby.

Manaster B. (2002b). Miscellaneous, including hematogenous disorders and infection. In Manaster, B. J., Disler, D. G., & May, D. A. (eds.). *Musculoskeletal imaging. The requisites.* 2nd ed. St. Louis: Mosby.

May, D., & Disler, D. (2002). Generalizations. In Manaster, B. J., Disler, D. G., & May, D. A. (eds.). *Musculoskeletal imaging. The requisites.* 2nd ed. St. Louis: Mosby.

May, D. A., Purins, J. L., & Smith, D. K. (1996). MR Imaging of occult traumatic fractures and muscular injuries of the hip and pelvis in elderly patients. *American Journal of Roentgenology, 166,* 1075–1078.

Millis, M. B., & Kocher, M. (2003). Hip and pelvic injuries in the young athlete. In DeLee, J. C., Drez, D., & Miller, M. (eds.). *DeLee & Drez's orthopedic sports medicine.* 2nd ed. Philadelphia: Saunders.

Mintz, D., Hooper, T, Connell, D., et al. (2005). Magnetic resonance imaging of the hip. Detection of labral and chondral abnormalities using noncontrast imaging. *Arthroscopy, 21,* 385–393.

Murphey, M. D., Andrews, C. L., Flemming, D. J., et al. (1996). Primary tumors of the spine: radiologic-pathologic correlation. *Radiographics, 16,* 1131–1158.

Murphy, W. A., & Preston, B. J. (2001). Joint disease. In Grainger, R. E., Allison, D., Adam, A., et al. *Grainger & Allison's diagnostic radiology: a textbook of medical imaging.* 4th ed. London, Churchill Livingstone.

Ogino, I, Okamato, N., Ong, Y, et al. (2003). Pelvic insufficiency fractures in postmenopausal women with advanced cervical cancer treated by radiotherapy. *Radiotherapy and Oncology, 68,* 61–67.

Oka, M., & Monu, J. (2004). Prevalence and patterns of occult hip fractures and mimics revealed by MRI. *American Journal of Roentgenology, 182,* 283–288.

Otte, M. T, Helms, C. A., & Fritz, R. C. (1997). MR imaging of supra-acetabular insufficiency fractures. *Skeletal Radiology, 26,* 279–283.

Overdeck, K., & Palmer, W. (2004). Imaging of the hip and groin injuries in athletes. *Seminars in Musculoskeletal Radiology, 8,* 41–55.

Ozonoff, M. B. (1992). The hip. In Bralow, L., ed. *Pediatric orthopedic radiology.* 2nd ed. Philadelphia: Saunders.

Plotz, G., Brossman, J., von Knoch M., et al. (2001). Magnetic resonance arthrography of the acetabular labrum: value of radial reconstructions. *Archives of Orthopaedic and Trauma Surgery, 121,* 450–457.

Priolo, F., & Cerase, A. (1998). The current role of radiography in the assessment of skeletal tumors and tumor-like lesions. *European Journal of Radiology, 27(*Suppl. 1), S77–85.

Reynolds, R. A. (1999). Diagnosis and treatment of slipped capital femoral epiphysis. *Current Opinions in Pediatrics, 111,* 80–83.

Scutellari, P. N., Addonisio, G., Righi, R., & Giganti, M. (2000). Diagnostic imaging of bone metastases. *Radiologica Medica (Torino), 100,* 429–435.

Stevens, M. A., El-Khoury, G. Y, Kathol, M, H., et al. (1999). Imaging features of avulsion injuries. *Radiographics, 19,* 655–672.

Smet, A. A., de. (1993). Magnetic resonance findings in skeletal muscle tears. *Skeletal Radiology, 22,* 479–484.

Soubrier, M., Dubost, JJ., Boisgard, S., et al. (2003). Insufficiency fracture. A survey of 60 cases and review of the literature. *Joint, Bone Spine: Revue du Rhumatisme, 70,* 209–18.

Steinberg, M. (1997). Avascular necrosis: diagnosis, staging, and management. *Journal of Musculoskeletal Medicine*, 14,13–25.

Sundaram, M. (2003). Imaging of metastatic bone disease. In El-Khoury, G. (ed.). *Essentials of musculoskeletal imaging*. Philadelphia: Churchill Livingstone.

Temmerman, O., Raijmakers, P., David, E., et al. (2004). A comparison of radiographic and scintigraphic techniques to assess aseptic loosening of the acetabular component in a total hip replacement. *Journal of Bone and Joint Surgery (American)*, 86, 2456–2463.

Theumann, N. H., Verdon, J. P., Mouhsine, E., et al. (2002). Traumatic injuries: imaging of pelvic fractures. *European Radiology*, 12, 312–1330.

Umans, N., Liebling, M. S., Moy, L., et al. (1998). Slipped capital femoral epiphysis: a physeal lesion diagnosed by MRI, with radiographic and CT correlation. *Skeletal Radiology*, 27, 139–144.

Verbeeten, K., Hermann, K., Hasselqvist, M., et al. (2005). The advantages of MRI in detection of occult hip fractures. *European Radiology*, 15, 165–169.

Vinson, E. N., & Major, N. M. (2003). MR imaging of ankylosing spondylitis. *Seminars in Musculoskeletal Radiology*, 7, 103–114.

Wall, E. (1999). Legg-Calvé-Perthes' disease. *Orthopedics*, 11, 76–79.

Weber, M., Hasler, P., & Gerber, H. (1993). Insufficiency fractures of the sacrum: twenty cases and review of the literature. *Spine*, 18, 2507–2512.

Wunderbaldinger, P., Bremer, C., Matuszewski, L., et al. (2001). Efficient radiological assessment of the internal snapping hip syndrome. *European Radiology*, 11, 1743–1747.

Yamamoto, Y., Hamada, Y., Ide, T., & Usui, I. (2005). Arthroscopic surgery to treat intra-articular type snapping hip. *Arthroscopy*, 21, 1120–1125.

Yamamoto, Y., Ide, T., Nakamura, M., et al. (2004). Arthroscopic partial limbectomy in hip joints with acetabular hypoplasia. *Arthroscopy*, 21, 586–591.

Yamamoto, T., Kubo, T, & Hirasawa, Y. (1999). A clinicopathologic study of transient osteoporosis of the hip. *Skeletal Radiology*, 28, 621–627.

Young, J. W. R., & Resnik, C. S. (1990). Fracture of the pelvis: current concepts of classification. *American Journal of Roentgenology*, 155, 1169–1175.

Yu, W., Feng, F., Dion, E., et al. (1998). Comparison of radiography, computed tomography and magnetic resonance imaging in the detection of sacroiliitis accompanying ankylosing spondylitis. *Skeletal Radiology*, 27, 27:311–320.

Yu, J. S. (2000). Hip and femur trauma. *Seminars in Musculoskeletal Radiology*, 4, 205–220.

Zelle, B., Gruen, G., Brown, S., & George, S. (2005). Sacroiliac joint dysfunction. Evaluation and management. *Clinical Journal of Pain*, 21, 446–455.

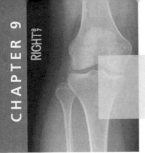

The Knee

Imaging of the knee has changed dramatically during the past 10 years as a result of enhanced imaging capabilities but also owing to a better appreciation of the pathology or injury, and thus planning of surgical intervention or other treatment. The primary challenges at the knee include multiple joints, weight-bearing functions, and a variety of anatomic structures. Because clinicians always attempt to gain the greatest assurance of detail, they have often accepted the use of magnetic resonance imaging (MRI) as requisite to models of "best practice." Importantly, the use of plain radiography coupled with appropriate physical examination provides very acceptable levels of sensitivity and specificity for most routine clinical examinations (O'Shea, 1996). The use of MRI is best applied in complex patients (multiple injuries) or where structural tissue differentiation is desired, particularly if surgical planning can be enhanced. The most common approach for MRI use is to use T1-weighted images to outline basic anatomic detail and T2-weighted images to better define specific structures (particularly soft and fibrous tissues) and to provide greater contrast. A very exciting evolution is to use additional modifications such as high-resolution proton density–fast spin echo (FSE) to elucidate and map articular cartilage changes which occur early in the "disease process" and thus permit clinicians hopefully to treat patients better based on predicted outcomes (Figure 9–1).

The knee joint proper (tibiofemoral joint) is divided into the medial and lateral compartments for evaluative processes. The medial compartment is larger and transmits more than half of the weight-bearing loads to the tibia, thus rendering it more susceptible to arthritic changes. This is coupled with the lateral compartment being less stable and allowing greater amounts of rotation. These actions are functionally defined by bony architecture as the medial side presents as a convex femur articulating with a concave tibia, whereas the convex lateral femoral condyle sits atop a flat or convex lateral tibia. The menisci sit between these opposing structures, enhancing the congruence or articulation and allowing better weight-bearing loads to be dispersed (greater area of contact, lesser per unit area of loading). The flexion/extension movements are controlled via both the bony articulation and the complex ligamentous structures while the musculature provides the ability to move but also to absorb and dissipate functional loading impacts. The musculature performs through the patellofemoral joint (patella and underlying femoral sulcus) in a pattern of motion controlled by both soft tissues (specific ligaments, capsule, and musculature) as well as the level of bony congruence and orientation of the patella with the sulcus. Specialized views are used to attempt to give data referring to these patterns with moderate success.

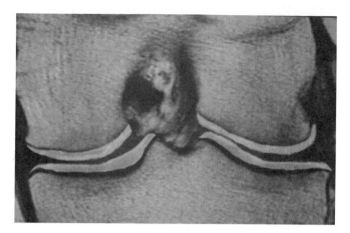

Figure 9–1 In this T2-weighted FSE technique, note the heterogeneous appearance of the signal from the articular cartilage weight-bearing area in the femoral condyle. Subtle changes of signal intensity can be indicative of early alterations in the functional status of the articular cartilage.

KNEE: STANDARD CONVENTIONAL RADIOGRAPHS

The initial screening views are traditionally the anteroposterior (AP) (supine or weight bearing) and supine or side-lying lateral views (Figures 9–2 and 9–3). These views allow evaluation of basic orientation (joint space and alignment [varus/valgus]) as well as the patellar position, bony contours, and congruity (observing obvious fractures), bone density (ruling out tumors), status of the epiphyseal plates, and obvious deformities or abnormal structure presentation. These views are nearly always used to rule out the obvious but combined with appropriate manual examination, provides a relatively impressive sensitivity and specificity to actual diagnosis. (O'Shea, 1996) Many clinicians substitute a 30-degree weight-bearing view rather than use the full-extension position as it frequently provides a better picture of functional contact between the joint surfaces (Figure 9–4). Another view that may be used during screening to better present the weight-bearing condylar surfaces and the intercondylar area of the femur is the intercondylar notch view (Figure 9–5). This intercondylar view shows early changes of the medial femoral condyle—osteonecrosis or dissecans-type lesion.

Fractures of the proximal tibia and distal femur are typically seen with the two or three standard views (Figure 9–6). The great challenge to the clinician is determining the best treatment approach whenever articular cartilage is involved or if the epiphyseal plate is disrupted in those that have not reached complete ossification (growth plate closure). Commonly used classification systems of the tibial plateau fractures link the type of fracture (depressed or the more clean split) to mechanism/force (valgus, varus, axial, rotation) and the resultant picture (e.g., split, depression, displaced, comminuted). A similar process is seen with distal femur fractures related to the condyles, with supracondylar, intercondylar, and condylar being the usual descriptors. When surgery is planned, surgeons will often obtain a computed tomographic (CT) image to better

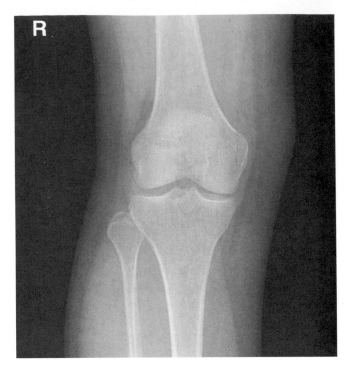

Figure 9–2 An AP radiograph of the knee allows for basic assessment of bone integrity and alignment. Note the superimposition of the patella over the distal femur.

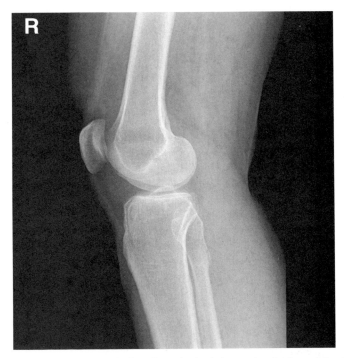

Figure 9–3 A lateral view radiograph also allows for basic inspection for bone integrity and alignment. The patella is better visualized in this view.

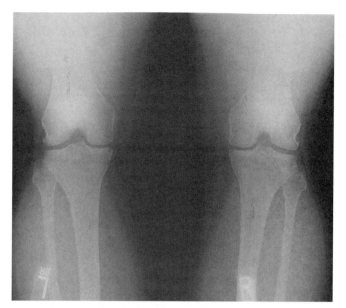

Figure 9–4 When involvement of the articular surfaces is suspected, a position of approximately 30 degrees of knee flexion while weight bearing is often used. This position allows for greater inspection of the relationship of the articular surfaces.

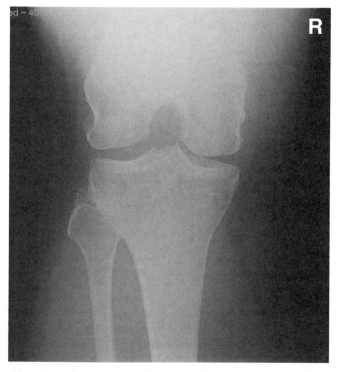

Figure 9–5 In this radiograph, an intercondylar or "notch" view is used to more closely inspect the femoral condyle articular surfaces.

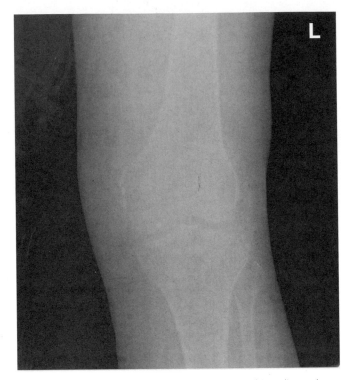

Figure 9–6 Findings of fractures are sometimes quite subtle. In this radiograph, one must inspect closely to find the fracture line extending through the lateral tibial plateau. Also note the lateral sub-luxation of the patella.

delineate the articular surface to facilitate appropriate fixation to provide optimal congruity (Figure 9–7). Surgeons have begun to be more aggressive in the use of better and stronger early fixation of these fractures as long-term results have not been consistently good with minimal fixation. Surgeons often will use substantial metal plates and fixators to give the best opportunity for good outcomes.

A greater challenge is present for the patellofemoral joint assessment as static positioning greatly limits the applicability to actual patient function and articular cartilage in reality is often a tissue of interest. Most orthopedists today place less importance on static images as normal radiographs often accompany the patient presenting with anterior knee pain. Since the patella moves over the underlying sulcus, many different radiographic positions have been designed to better display meaningfully these essentially tangential relationships as well as actual descriptive measurement processes (e.g., sulcus angle, congruence, q-angle, a-angle). The classic initial patellar radiograph is known as a "skyline or sunrise" view. This film was often done at 90 degrees of flexion but is more commonly performed with lesser amounts of flexion to better demonstrate the seating of the patella within the femoral sulcus (Figure 9–8). Seating of the patellae is shown allowing right to left comparison as well as actual orientation. Various techniques have been espoused, with the main features being angle of knee flexion, position of

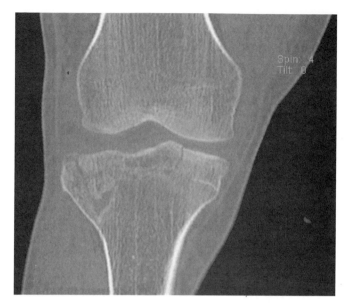

Figure 9–7 This coronal slice CT image reveals detail of the tibial plateau fracture not appreciable by radiography. Such detail is particularly useful in surgical decision making.

cassette, and direction/focus of beam. These views include the Hughston (prone & 55 degrees), Merchant (supine and 45 degrees), and Laurin (sitting and 20 degrees) (Hughston et al., 1984; Fulkerson, 2004). The key factor is the clinical attempt of discerning the orientation of patella to sulcus and the actual shape of patellar facets as they articulate. Although the Wiberg Classification scheme is the most commonly used to

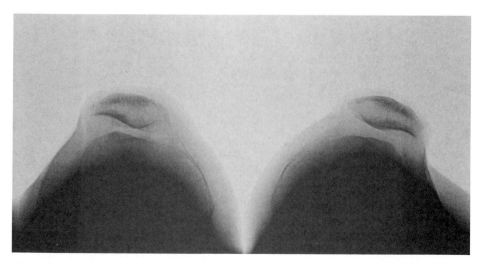

Figure 9–8 In this bilateral sunrise or skyline view, note the difference in positioning of the patellae. The image on the right shows much more lateral positioning.

describe patellar shape (axial morphology), it is again important to accept its correlation to function being limited (Wiberg, 1941). In the recent past, CT and functional MRI have been applied to these patients but with limited success. Clinicians are faced with acceptance that the complexity of patellar motion also includes the movement or positioning of the underlying sulcus (particularly during closed chain–weight-bearing functional tasks), and that the representation achieved with imaging does not necessarily provide the desired answer to the clinical problem.

As the patella represents the largest sesamoid in the body and has a prominent exposed position, it is vulnerable to fractures via external impacts or compression. These fractures are often described or classified by overall appearance or orientation (vertical, transverse, or comminuted). These fractures are normally elucidated well with a normal knee series of plain radiographs (Figure 9–9). The patella may also have injuries associated

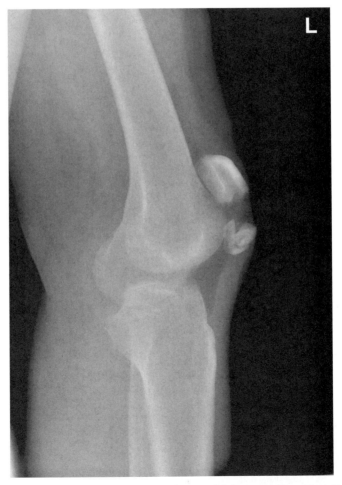

Figure 9–9 This lateral view radiograph reveals a clear patellar fracture with marked displacement of the fracture fragments.

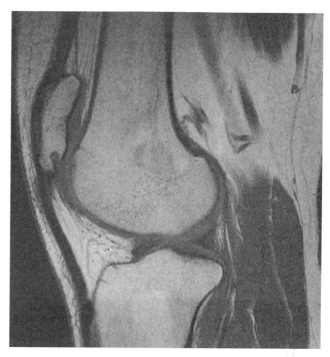

Figure 9–10 In addition to the patella alta present, note the sequelae of partial or attempted avulsion of the pole of the patella in this image. The posterior surface of the patella also suggests considerable chondromalacia.

with the loading associated with high eccentric muscle activations in the middle portion of the range of motion (tension loads resulting in a transverse fracture). These are typically described as "avulsion injuries" and more commonly result in changes at the ligament insertion rather than within the patella itself (Figure 9–10). When they are at the patellar insertion, they are known as Sinding-Larsen-Johansson disease or jumpers knee, while Osgood-Schlatter disease is the descriptor at the tibial tuberosity. Superior and inferior to the patella, quadriceps tendon and patellar ligament avulsion/rupture, respectively, do occur; again typically with high eccentric muscle activation, as seen in a single leg landing from a jump. Complete rupture of the restraint either provides a patella that moves with quadriceps activation superiorly without generating knee extension or a patella that will remain stationary when attempted quadriceps activation occurs; again without the expected knee extension. Occasionally, a bipartite patella will be discovered incidentally (Figures 9–11A & B).

 ## SOFT TISSUE STRUCTURES OF THE KNEE

The unique weight-bearing surfaces of the femoral–tibial joint require strong ligamentous support and control to permit normal function. Likewise, the joint loading is such that meniscal structures are present to better distribute axial loads to the articular surfaces.

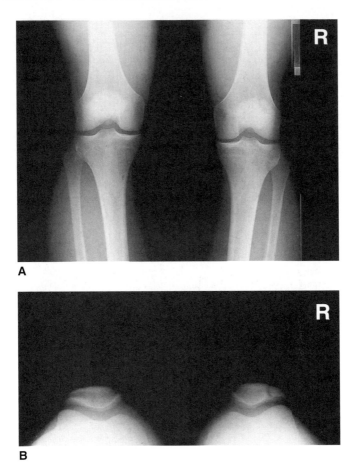

A

B

Figure 9–11 In these two conventional radiographs from the (A) AP and (B) sunrise views, respectively. A bipartite patella is revealed as an incidental finding.

These structures are thus at risk with weight-bearing activities, particularly weight bearing with rotation. The MRI has become the gold standard for these assessments with very high sensitivity and specificity for structural delineation. It should noted that MRI should ideally be employed to determine tissue involvement and surgical planning when standard films or clinical assessment are not definitive. Typically, ligamentous damage is strongly correlated to the mechanism of injury and high suspicion accompanies patient presentation. Reliance on this modality is expensive and can be seen as unnecessarily adding to expenditures. A good thought process is always to consider: Will the results of this assessment change the way we are going to treat this patient? If the answer is no, restraint may be appropriate.

Through the multiple views the MRI allows identification of the four primary ligaments (medial and lateral collaterals and anterior and posterior cruciates), the shape and densities of the medial and lateral menisci (type of tear and location can often be ascertained), as well as the volume and types of fluids present in the joint (Figures 9–12 to 9–14). It also provides a picture of the fat pad and capsular/bursal outlines again

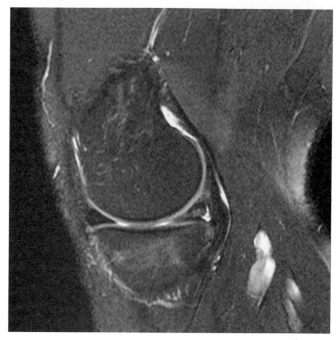

Figure 9–12 This sagittal slice MRI reveals increased signal intensity in the posterior horn of the meniscus as well as at the meniscocapsular junction, suggesting a tear of the meniscus and possible separation from the peripheral attachment.

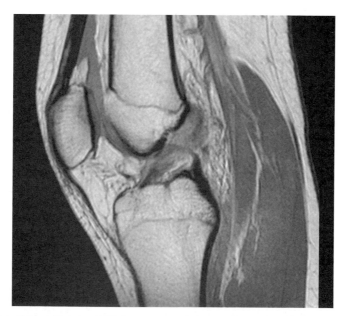

Figure 9–13 In this sagittal view MRI slice, rupture of the anterior cruciate ligament is demonstrated approximating the tibial attachment. This image is from a 16-year-old female; note the incompletely closed epiphyseal plates.

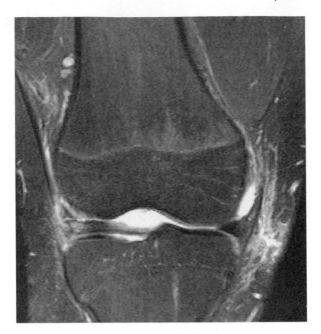

Figure 9–14 In this coronal slice MR image, areas of increased signal intensity are noted in the medial and lateral collateral ligaments, suggesting incomplete tears of each. Also note the appearance of the lateral meniscus; the increased signal intensity in the body of the meniscus is consistent with a tear of this structure.

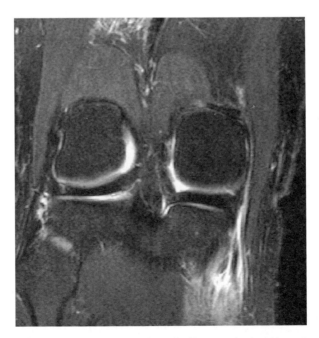

Figure 9–15 This coronal slice MR image reveals marked increase in signal intensity and suggestions of discontinuity of the semitendinosus at its myotendinous junction and its tibial attachment. Such findings are consistent with a nearly complete tear.

related to fluid volumes while defining the extensor mechanism (quadriceps musculature and insertions to the patella through to the tibial tuberosity via the patellar tendon/ ligament). Thus, injury to musculotendinous units can also be delineated with the soft tissue capabilities of MRI (Figure 9–15). It easy to see how today nearly all patients with significant trauma or if reconstructive ligament surgery is planned will have an MRI assessment.

DEGENERATIVE CONDITIONS AND UNIQUE KNEE CONDITIONS

Osteoarthritis (OA) is one of the most common conditions seen at the knee, with a very significant portion of the population over the age of 60 having some level of this present. Imaging studies demonstrate the hallmark later changes associated with these patients (increased bone density and osteophytes, changes in shape/contours/orientations, and loss of joint space). Imaging is more limited in the early phases as bone changes are later, but abnormal alignment and previous injury may predispose one to developing significant OA requiring treatment (Figures 9–16A & B). Early treatment focuses on

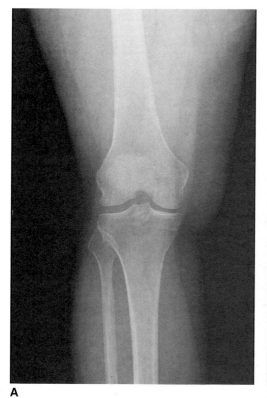
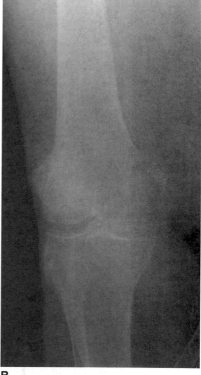

A   B

Figure 9–16 A. In this AP radiograph, there is very early indication of a loss of medial compartment joint space, which is consistent with early OA. **B.** In this image, the degenerative disease process is advanced as evidenced by the near complete obliteration of medial joint space, sclerosis of the subchondral bone, flattening of the medial femoral condyle, and osteophyte formation around the margin of the tibia.

pain/inflammation control and strengthening. When OA is long standing, many patients will receive a total knee replacement, with the vast majority enjoying a very positive outcome (Figure 9–17). Surgeons typically improve the alignment of the tibia and femur during the implantation, which minimizes future abnormal loading to better provide long-term function.

Ostechondritis dissecans is an articular detachment which includes an attached piece of underlying bone, thus creating an osteochondral fracture or flap. It is thought that these are probably related to an impact injury (but actual causation is unknown), there is a stronger prevalence in young men than women, and the lesion location is most commonly the femoral condyles (particularly the medial condyle). Plain films are helpful in large lesions and when separation has occurred (Figure 9–18), but MRI is better when more definitive articular surface assessment is required. Treatment is predicated on lesion size, location, and relationship to underlying bone (attached and in situ, partially attached, hinged, floating freely) (Figures 9–19A & B).

MRI also provides information concerning injury within the trabecular bone as evidenced by the appearance of marrow edema (Figure 9–20), which typically occurs in response to inordinate loading, either in macrotrauma or in some microtrauma circumstances.

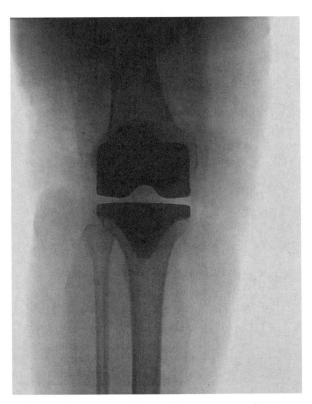

Figure 9–17 This radiograph demonstrates the metallic components of the knee prosthesis and the joint space provided by the polyethylene spacer.

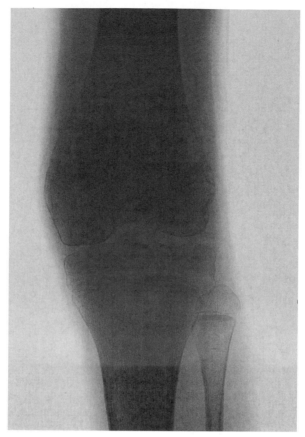

Figure 9–18 Observe the irregularity in the normal convexity of the medial femoral condyle in this AP conventional radiograph. Although not confirmatory, this finding along with the remainder of the clinical picture is strongly indicative of osteochondritis dessicans. Also note the incompletely closed epiphyseal plates typical of the population of patients in which this disorder becomes symptomatic.

 ## CLINICAL RELEVANCE TO PHYSICAL THERAPY

Rehabilitation Implications 1

The patient was a 46-year-old male ex-athlete (collegiate football linemen). He is 6 feet 4 inches tall and weighs 260 lb. His chief complaint of was medial knee pain that was particularly associated with tennis. Orthopedic evaluation demonstrated posterior medial joint line pain. There was minimal swelling that had become recurrent over the past few months. It was often associated with playing a significant amount of tennis as in participating in a weekend tournament. The clinical picture was suggestive of a medial meniscus tear. The plain films were negative, while the MRI was positive for a posterior medial meniscus tear. The orthopedic surgeon performed an arthroscopic evaluation, but was

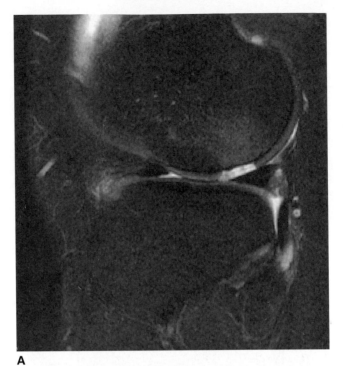

A

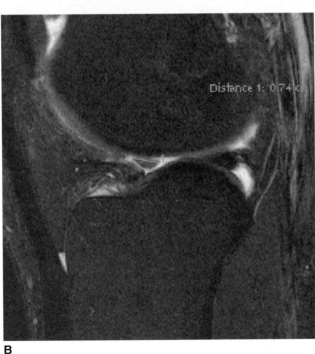

B

Figure 9–19 A. In this sagittal slice MR image, the area of increased signal intensity along the articular surface of the femoral condyle is consistent with a chondral defect. Also note immediately subjacent to this defect, the subtle increase of signal intensity consistent with marrow edema. **B.** In this image of the same patient, the radiologist has located and electronically measured the loose body chondral fragment from the defect in the prior image.

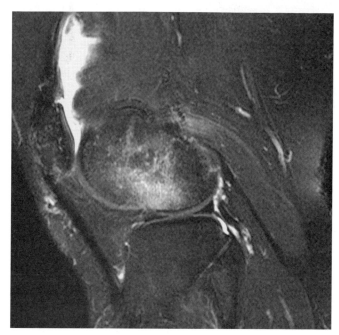

Figure 9–20 An area of marked increase of signal intensity within the femoral condyle is consistent with marrow edema. Also note the irregularity of the femoral condyle and the discontinuity of the signal of the articular cartilage. These findings are consistent with an impact fracture. The other particularly outstanding feature of this image is the large area of increased signal intensity in the suprapatellar pouch, which is a hallmark of joint effusion.

not able to find a tear in the medial meniscus. Approximately 9 months after the index procedure, the patient experienced a locking and giving way sensation of the knee. He was unable to achieve full extension without pain and thus presented with an antalgic gait. During the second arthroscopic procedure, the medial meniscus exhibited a posterior tear that now extended to the surface of the meniscus.

Clinical Pearls

Meniscal evaluation and treatment is difficult as (1) the tissue is fibrocartilaginous, (2) has a limited blood supply, (3) has limited neurologic innervation, and (4) is important in weight-bearing distribution and articular cartilage protection. Although the patient is an ex-athlete, one should not necessarily expect meniscal lesions associated with those activities. The greatest problem with ex-athletes is when they had significant injury to joint restraints while participating: they are at greatly increased risk of developing future problems, whereas those who did not experience injury are not necessarily at increased risk. (Although his weight of 260 lb is not helpful!) The clinical evaluative tests are quite limited, particularly in their specificity with single-leg rotational weight bearing being the most sensitive and specific test available. Joint line tenderness is typically helpful but limited in defining location—medial joint line tenderness may reflect lateral meniscal pathology.

It is interesting to note that this diagnosis was often provided by radiologists as there was abnormal signal in the medial meniscus. Unfortunately for the surgeon, this was representing intrasubstance degeneration that was not necessarily extending to the surface Communication between the radiologist and surgeon has better defined this process, but a significant challenge is present: Patients want *the* answer, and definitive surgery (as in fix it!) is perceived as the expected. It is difficult to convince patients to wait and see if they believe they can be fixed.

Rehabilitation Implications 2

The patient was a 22-year-old senior football wide receiver who complained of pain "shooting/burning into his leg" while participating in summer practices. The team was practicing two or three times daily, and his pain was associated with the act of getting into and accelerating out of a three-point stance (knee flexion with the hand placed onto the ground). The athlete reiterated that this happens every year during two-a-days

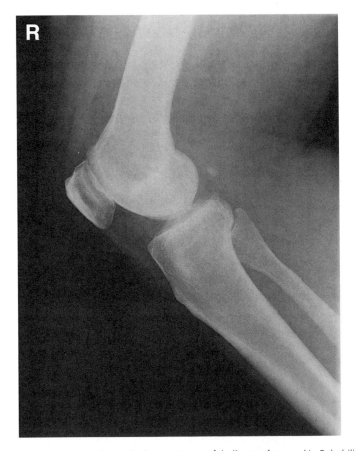

Figure 9–21 This lateral view radiograph demonstrates a fabella as referenced in Rehabilitation Implications 2. Often, a fabella is an incidental finding, but can occasionally be the source of symptoms.

(referring to summer preseason practice). Physical examination demonstrated tenderness to digital pressure over the lateral gastrocnemius (particularly with knee flexion), and a palpable structure within the muscle was present. Plain film radiography demonstrated a large fabella which corresponded to the area of concern. It was interesting to be able to duplicate his pain through the position and muscle activations associated with the specific tasks. The athlete then informed us again that it only bothers him getting into and out of the three-point stance during the second and third practice sessions. Also, he could do everything fine out of a standing posture or upright stance. We gave the head coach the recommendation to allow this athlete to run his routes out of the upright stance rather than the deeper flexion required of the three-point stance that was causing significant pain. The coach wanted that the athlete still to use the three-point stance as "he needs to practice like he plays." Fortunately, we were able to get the coach to compromise and have the athlete use the three-point stance only when doing live drills (scrimmage activities) and allowing the upright position for general practices during the second and or third sessions during the remainder of the preseason practices.

Clinical Pearl

The fabella (L. *little bean*) is an incidental finding the majority of the time (Figure 9–21). However, for this individual, performing significant knee flexion and then concentric muscle activation allowed a large cartilagenous fabella to place pressure on the peroneal nerve. The athlete was able not only to duplicate the pain-causing action, he had found a methodology which minimized it! A wise orthopedist is one who recognizes they don't treat x-rays and they must listen to the patient as they know the answers better than any of us.

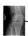 **REFERENCES**

Hughston, J. C, Walsh, W. M., & Puddu, G. (1984). *Patellar subluxation and dislocation*. Philadelphia: Saunders.

Fulkerson, J. P. (2004). *Disorders of the patellfemoral joint*. 4th ed. Baltimore: Williams & Wilkins.

O'Shea KJ, Murphy KP, Heekin RD, Herzwurm PJ. (1996). The diagnostic accuracy of history, physical examination, and radiographs in the evaluation of traumatic knee disorders. *Am Journ Sports Med, 24*, 2:164–167.

Wiberg, G. (1941). Roentgenographic and anatomic studies on the femoro-patellar joint. *Acta Orthopaedica Scandinavica, 12*, 319–410.

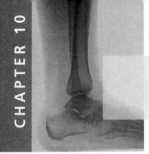
The Ankle and Foot

Since the ankle complex serves as the transition from the "leg" to the foot, significant forces are placed through these structures resulting in frequent injuries. The talus sits between the medial and lateral malleoli within what is described as the ankle mortise. The orientation of the mortise (lateral malleolus more distal and posterior than the medial) dictates the motion of plantar flexion to have an inversion component, while dorsiflexion includes eversion. As the lower extremity internally rotates during ambulation and the foot must be able to be placed onto the surface, the next inferior linkage to the foot provides a mechanism for dissipation of rotation (subtalar joint) while enabling the foot to adapt to uneven surfaces (serving as a mobile adaptor). It is obvious that a variety of ligamentous structures are required to control the bony structures and to interface with the muscular units permitting normal function. The osseous–ligamentous structures are shown in Figure 10–1A & B, respectively, in medial and lateral orientations. These relationships have been described at length by Inman (1976). It is interesting to note how Inman used models to explain the intricate interrelationships and how the ankle must be viewed as apart of the overall complex. This can be perceived as enabling the lower extremity to perform required "functional" tasks while permitting the foot to transfer weight-bearing loads. Unfortunately, the large loads and unique triplanar action of these structures does predispose them to injury.

 ## ANKLE

Standard Plain Radiographs

The initial views are the traditional anteroposterior (AP) and lateral following the 90 Degree Rule (Figures 10–2 and 10–3). When the orientation of the talar dome in the mortise is in question, a mortise view is performed (Figure 10–4). Some clinicians prefer what is described as an oblique view ,which is somewhat more effective in delineating malleolar relationships (Figure 10–5). Clinicians will typically see an "ankle series" including an AP, lateral, and either the mortise or oblique. It is very interesting to note that the routine use of the ankle series has come under question as a set of manual palpations and clinical observations appear to be sufficient to rule out fractures when applied by therapists or surgeons (Stiell et al., 1994).

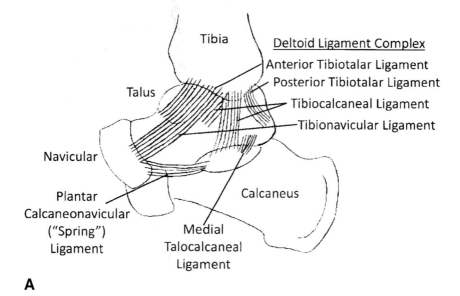

Figure 10–1 Ankle ligaments. **A.** Medial view **B.** Lateral view.

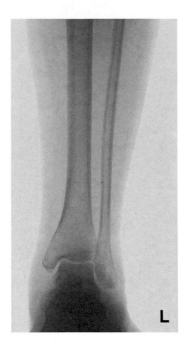

Figure 10–2 A normal-appearing AP view radiograph of the ankle. Note the slight overlap of the tibia and fibula at the distal articulation.

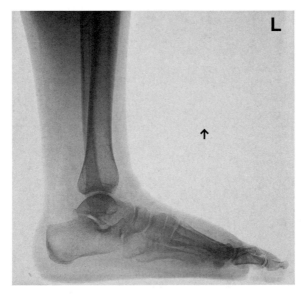

Figure 10–3 A normal-appearing lateral view radiograph of the ankle. Apparent in this view is not only the general osseous alignment but also the joint space of the talocrural joint.

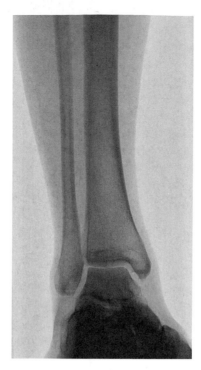

Figure 10–4 In this mortise view radiograph, the overlap of the distal tibia and fibula is eliminated, allowing for better visualization of the talus within the mortise.

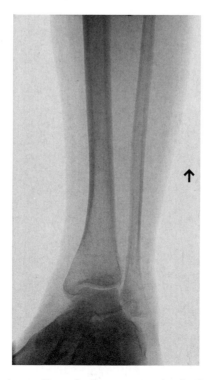

Figure 10–5 The oblique view radiograph allows greater visualization of the malleoli and their surrounding structures.

Special Plain Radiographic Views

In specific clinical presentations, additional views may be used to define bony problems. One of the more common needs in athletic populations includes evaluation of impingement , both anterior and posterior. These views are of the lateral nature with either complete plantar flexion (Figure 10–6) or dorsiflexion (Figure 10–7). The posterior problems are seen in dancers as their intense weight-bearing postures in the extremes of the range of motion place them at risk, while anterior problems occur in kicking sports.

Weight-bearing films are used to examine articular cartilage/joint space height and the distal tibiofibular relationship (syndesmosis). The articular cartilage/joint space film is typically a standing lateral (Figure 10–8). The loss of joint space and increased bone density commonly implies long-standing disease with considerable bony reaction. The syndesmosis view is done with weight bearing and dorsiflexion. The opening of the space between the tibia and fibula is examined but is often relatively minimally altered unless an additional stress is applied (Figure 10–9). This leads to the use of a non–weight-bearing stress test to the medial ligamentous structures (deltoid ligament) to assess if the

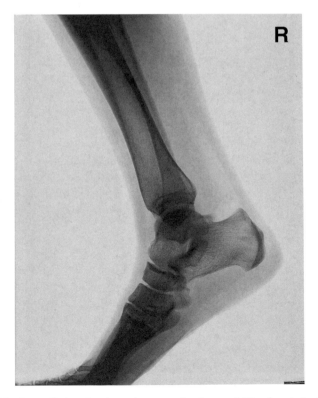

Figure 10–6 This plantar flexion view is used to assess for the possibility of posterior impingement at the talocrural joint by the relationship of the distal posterior tibia and posterior talus.

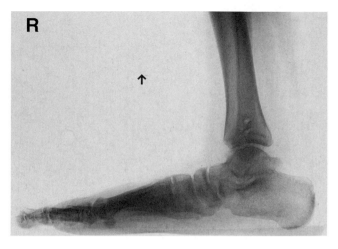

Figure 10–7 Similar to the plantar flexion view, the relationships of the anterior distal tibia and anterior talus are better appreciated in this dorsiflexion view.

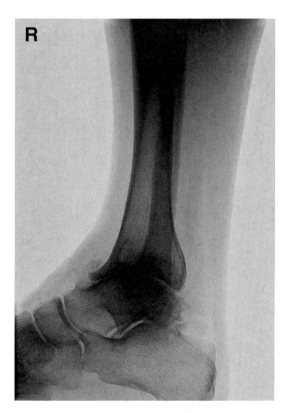

Figure 10–8 In this lateral weight-bearing view, note the increased opacity of the articular surfaces and loss of joint space, which is consistent with degenerative changes of the talocrural joint. Close inspection also reveals osteophyte formation about the joint margins.

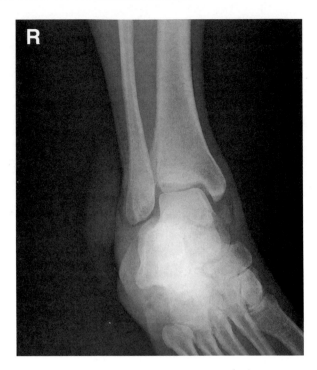

Figure 10–9 In this radiograph, note the increased space between the articular surfaces of the talus, tibia, and fibula, suggesting disruption of the mortise.

fibula will move laterally as well as the talus moving from the tibia. Long- standing diastasis (widening of the fibula from the tibia) is seen and can result in calcification of the tibiofibular ligament and development of osteoarthritic changes. Acute injuries to these structures normally occur with dorsiflexion and eversion stress through weight bearing, and do require a much longer rehabilitation than the very common lateral ligament sprains. Clinicians are able to palpate for tenderness anteriorly along this "space" with distance of tenderness proximally from the talus reflective of the severity of injury (small distance less serious than several centimeters of tenderness).

Fractures of the fibula may accompany the diastasis with the classic fracture being the Maisonneuve fracture. This combination includes the opening of the tibiofibular space and the medial talus-malleolar space and a resultant proximal fibular fracture (Figure 10–10). Classically, the fibular fracture is in the proximal third, but more liberally interpreted distal location has been accepted by many. Frequently, a medial malleolar fracture is also part of this complex.

Several other fractures are more difficult to evaluate as the symptoms are not nearly as well defined and palpable. These include fractures of the talus (particularly the talar dome) and are often missed on plain films. One of the clinical pearls of working with

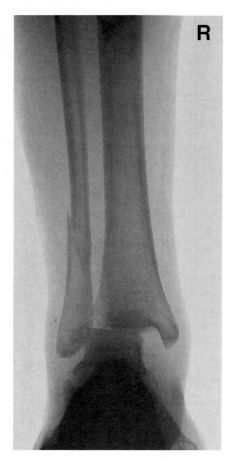

Figure 10–10 In this AP radiograph, disruption of the mortise and a fracture of the fibula are apparent. The mechanism of injury is usually due to an external rotation force. So-called Maisonneuve fractures are typically characterized by a proximal fibula fracture, although more distal injuries are sometimes included in this same category.

these patients is to request additional evaluation when symptoms continue for several weeks after initial "impact" injury. When weight-bearing activities continue to be symptomatic look for talar involvement.

Stress fractures are not very common at the ankle but can be seen at the distal fibula (runner's fracture) and the distal tibia (Figure 10–11). Plain film expression of bony reaction often takes several weeks and lags the patient presentation of pain with activity.

The last frequently used plain films of the ankle are stress views to evaluate the medial or lateral ligamentous structures, often described as "talar tilt." Because the medial complex (deltoid ligaments) is significantly stronger than the lateral ligaments (anterior talofibular, calcaneofibular, and posterior talofibular ligaments), lateral injuries with plantar flexion and inversion are much more common (Figures 10–12A & B).

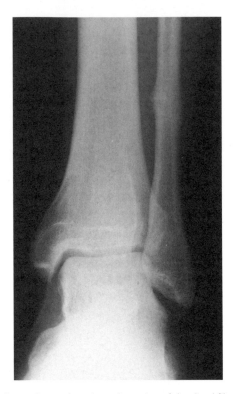

Figure 10–11 This AP radiograph reveals periosteal reaction of the distal fibula consistent with a stress fracture. Such injuries are often found in runners.

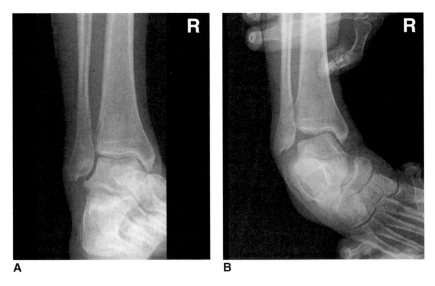

Figure 10–12 In the static, unstressed view (A), the alignment suggests little change from normal. The stress view (B), however, with passive positioning reveals marked opening of the mortise. This finding is indicative of significant injury of the lateral ligamentous structures, which would normally restrain this motion.

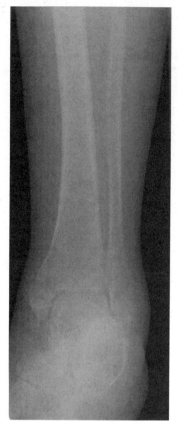

Figure 10–13 Fracture lines are apparent through both malleoli in this radiograph. Bimalleolar fractures typically occur from traumatic torsional forces.

Individuals who suffer traumatic injuries are subsequently likely to be seen by the rehabilitation professional, including those patients with bimalleolar fractures (Figure 10–13) in which the distal portions of the tibia and fibula are fractured. Although not a true malleolus, if the posterior aspect of the distal tibia is also affected, the injury is often referred to as a trimalleolar fracture (Figure 10–14).

 SPECIAL IMAGING

Computerized Tomography Scans
Tomography often enables delineation of cortical and trabecular orientations of bone better than plain films. A good example of its use at the ankle is in evaluation of talar dome injury (Figure 10–15). On plain film, it is difficult to see "surface" injury, which is more obvious through computed tomography (CT). This is an important test in patients when they exhibit weight-bearing pain that is persistent beyond the normal ankle sprain period of a few days.

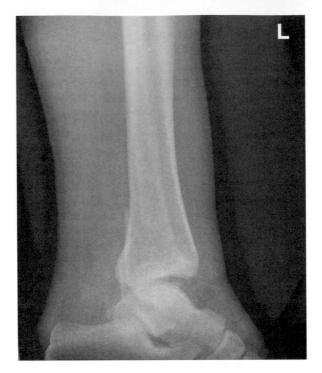

Figure 10–14 A third fracture line through the posterior distal tibia results in a so-called trimalleolar fracture as visualized in this lateral view. In addition to torsional forces, a supinatory force is also frequently suggested to occur with these injuries.

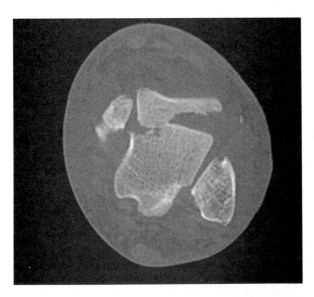

Figure 10–15 This CT axial slice of the talocrural joint reveals details of a talar dome fracture unlikely to be visualized by radiography. Determining the number and location of bone fragments is particularly helpful in surgical planning.

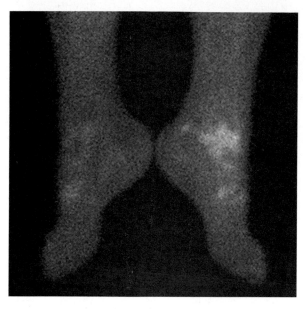

Figure 10–16 This scintigraphic image demonstrates increased isotope uptake within the ankle, particularly the talus. For this particular patient, a diagnosis of osteomyelitis was eventually confirmed.

Isotopic Bone Scans

The bone scan at the ankle is used in suspected stress fractures and to highlight areas of increased metabolic activity. The bone scan is often positive in stress fractures when the plain film is not, particularly in early evaluations. Increased uptake of the isotope is evident with metabolic changes as seen in Figure 10–16; in this case consistent with osteomyelitis.

Magnetic Resonance Imaging

Magnetic Resonance Imaging (MRI) at the ankle is used to examine soft tissue and osteochondral lesions. An excellent example is again the talar dome as seen in Figure 10–17. MRI can be used for soft tissue injury diagnosis, such as ligamentous injury (Figure 10–18), but is usually not required in normal circumstances related to cost and clinical assessment being sufficient.

Ultrasonography

Ultrasound use at the ankle allows tendon and cyst evaluation (Figure 10–19). The use of ultrasound is somewhat user dependent. However, because it is relatively inexpensive and effective, its use is expected to increase in the future.

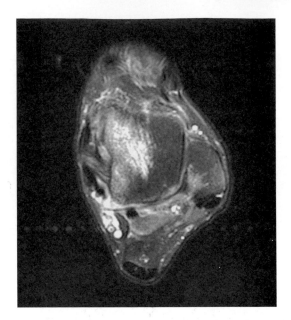

Figure 10–17 This axial MRI slice shows dramatically increased signal intensity at the talar dome consistent with an inflammatory response from osteochondral injury at the articular surface and below.

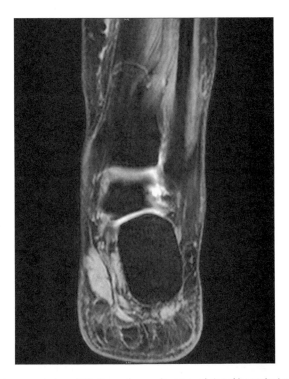

Figure 10–18 In this coronal plane MRI slice, a focus of increased signal intensity is present at the talus-fibula articulation. This finding is suggestive of inflammatory response within the posterior talofibular ligament, which is indicative of a partial tear.

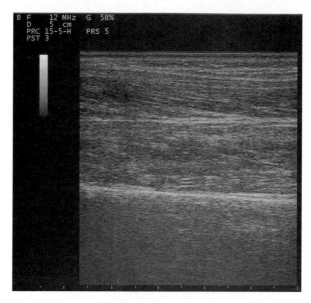

Figure 10–19 This image of the tendo calcaneus reveals continuity of the planes of tissue and consistency of signal within the tendon, which is typical of a normal tendon.

 ## THE FOOT

The foot provides the actual linkage to the support surface. It structurally must be able to adapt to uneven surfaces while enabling the constant changes associated with weight bearing to propulsion to free movement to preparing for weight bearing. This is accomplished through the foot having a longitudinal arch and medial/lateral arch. These arches are supported and reinforced by numerous ligaments and muscle–tendon units.

The osseous structures are often divided into functional units: hindfoot (talus and calcaneus), midfoot (navicular, cuboid, and cuneiforms), and forefoot (metatarsals and phalanges). A vast number of ligaments and capsules are associated with these segments. It is important to recognize how effectively these functions occur in the normal individual but also how predictable the alterations in function result in injury, reaction, or disability.

Standard Plain Radiography

The standard foot "series" is the AP, lateral, and oblique. The AP view is a dorsal to plantar with the foot placed on the cassette (Figure 10–20). Note that the first and second toes are longer than the remaining toes; thus, assuring the medial weight-bearing loads are distributed appropriately. The lateral view is taken with the medial side of the foot on the cassette, while the oblique is a view with the lateral side of the foot raised approximately 30 degrees off the cassette (from the AP position) (Figure 10–21). The AP and lateral follow the 90 Degree Rule, while the oblique is designed to better display the

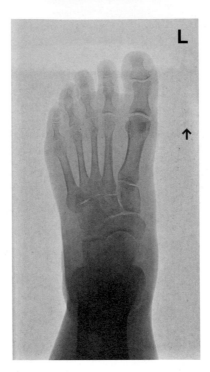

Figure 10–20 From this AP radiograph of the foot, general bone integrity and alignment may be evaluated.

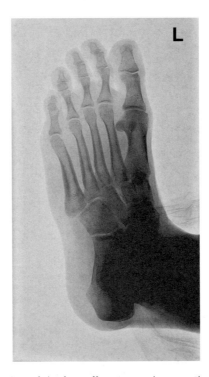

Figure 10–21 The oblique view of the foot offers perspective sometimes obscured by overlapping layers of osseous tissue from the lateral view.

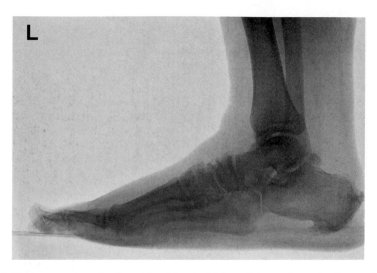

Figure 10–22 An osteophyte (heel spur) is evident in this lateral view radiograph. The spur is typically an indication of response to repeated stresses applied at this region and is not directly the problem.

"anterior structures" (metatarsals and phalanges). This series can be augmented with other plain films when special clinical data present.

One of the common problems seen in the foot is plantar fasciitis, with the typical presentation of severe "heel pain," particularly with the initial weight-bearing step in the morning. The lateral view frequently shows a heel spur, but it has very little clinical significance. Many patients will present with unilateral fasciitis but bilateral heel spurs. Figure 10–22 demonstrates the common findings as well as the additional changes seen in chronic cases.

Special Plain Radiographic Views

Weight-bearing views can be used particularly when questions of alignment are the clinical focus. One of the most common diagnoses is hallux valgus (angulation of the first metatarsophalangeal joint). Figure 10–23 demonstrates the expected loss of alignment in these patients. A less severe problem occurs on the lateral forefoot when the fifth metatarsophalangeal veers into a varus position resulting in a bunionette (Figure 10–24). Another common disorder is the hammer or claw toe deformity (Figure 10–25). Surgeries are common for these patients, if shoe adjustments are unable to prevent ongoing pressure.

Fractures of the foot are relatively common. Acute fractures are usually relatively easily viewed as the injury mechanism and bony tenderness alerts the clinician. One of the special groups of fractures is to the base of the fifth metatarsal. These injuries are typically classified as either transverse (proximal fifth), Jones' (more distal transverse fracture), or spiral. The Jones fracture is often very difficult to treat successfully, with the final result often being a nonunion. Figure 10–26 demonstrates a nondisplaced proximal fracture with greater delineation by CT (Figure 10–27).

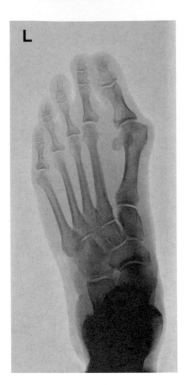

Figure 10–23 Deformity along the first ray of the foot consistent with hallux valgus is apparent on this AP radiograph of the foot.

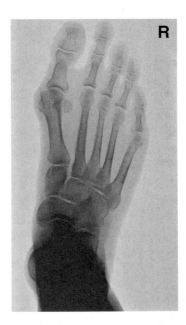

Figure 10–24 In this AP radiograph of the foot, varus deformity at the fifth metatarsophalangeal joint is evident, which consistent with a developing bunionette.

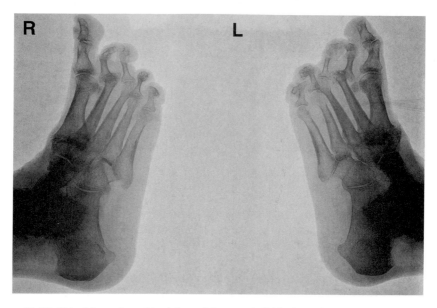

Figure 10–25 This oblique view of both feet of the same individual reveals multiple gross deformities including hammer and claw toes.

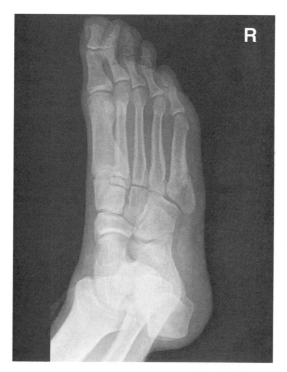

Figure 10–26 Fractures of the fifth metatarsal are relatively common. In this oblique view of the foot, one must look closely to find the fracture line at the base of the fifth metatarsal.

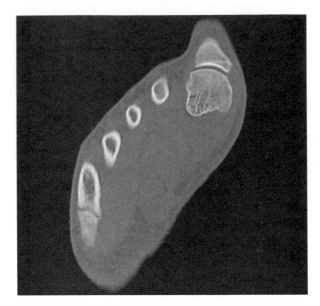

Figure 10–27 Greater detail by CT of the fifth metatarsal reveals a more apparent fracture line. Close inspection demonstrates subtle suggestions of sclerosis along the fracture line, which is consistent with nonunion.

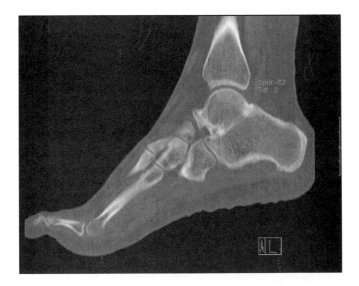

Figure 10–28 This sagittal slice CT demonstrates two particular areas of concern along the articular surfaces of the talus and calcaneus, which is consistent with a coalition.

Stress fractures of the metatarsals are common in forced overuse environments (e.g., military training, athletic practices, dancing). Plain films will often provide information on stress fractures but often follows a time lag with symptoms before detection. Navicular stress fractures do occur particularly in runners. They are best appreciated through bone scan and CT follow-up if positive.

Special Imaging

Computerized Tomography Scans

CT in the foot can be used to delineate the articular surfaces in the joints with Figure 10–28 showing this vividly. Since most of the foot can be accessed through the normal 90 Degree Rule, plain films are often sufficient except in areas of significant overlap (most often in the hindfoot or midfoot). For greater detail, however, CT offers the clinician more comprehensive visualization of the possible pathology. In Figure 10–29, a comminuted fracture of the calcaneus is more fully appreciated than it would be on conventional radiography. Occasionally, more sophisticated imaging is required as demonstrated by recently developed three-dimensional CT (Figures 10–30A & B).

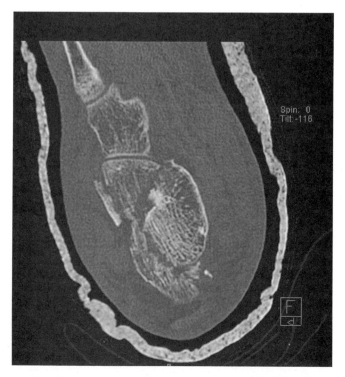

Figure 10–29 An axial slice CT of the calcaneus not only has diagnostic value in detecting a fracture, but the extent of the fracture to comminution and displacement of the fragments is well shown.

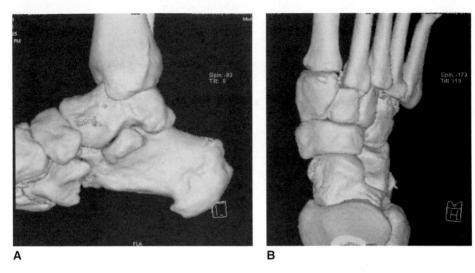

A   B

Figure 10–30 Remarkable detail can be revealed in these normal-appearing three-dimensional CT images of the talocalcaneal joint (A), and the tarsus (B), respectively.

Isotopic Bone Scan

Bone scans can be used to detect early stress fractures with increased isotope uptake corresponding to overuse history and symptoms. The bone scan will be positive several weeks prior to plain films showing stress reaction.

Magnetic Resonance Imaging

MRI also has the ability to detect bony changes such as stress responses and fractures prior to detection on conventional radiography as suggested in Figure 10–31. The greatest contribution of MRI has been to delineate soft tissue problems. In directly visualizing soft tissue continuity as well as markers of inflammatory response, MRI is capable of providing information to assist in clarifying sometimes complex clinical presentations. Figure 10–32 demonstrates injury to tendinous structures in remarkable detail.

Ultrasound Imaging

Ultrasonography has been used to examine tendons and other soft tissues such as bursae. Discontinuity of the signal is suggestive of significant tissue injury.

 CLINICAL RELEVANCE TO PHYSICAL THERAPY

Rehabilitation Implications

A 21-year-old intercollegiate basketball player presented with an acute ankle sprain. His mechanism of injury was plantar flexion/inversion associated with stepping on an opponent's foot. He had a positive anterior drawer (indicating a third-degree injury of the anterior talofibular ligament) but a negative talar tilt (calcaneofibular ligament was intact).

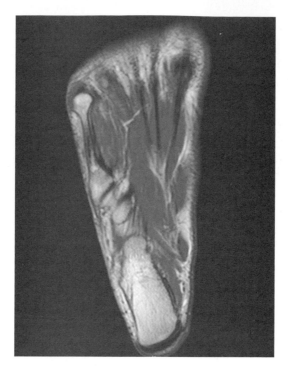

Figure 10–31 A stress response is evident in the diaphysis of the fifth metatarsal in this image. Detection of such injury may be particularly valuable in clinical decision making in the absence of overt fracture.

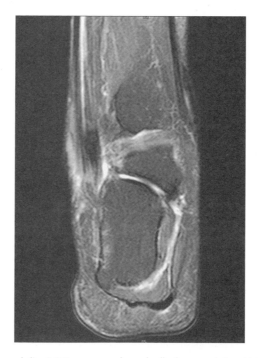

Figure 10–32 This coronal slice MR image reveals markedly decreased signal intensity in the peroneus longus and brevis tendons, which is consistent with tears in both structures.

Because he was a high-profile athlete, a plain ankle series was done with no positive findings. Over the next 2 weeks, he received the normal PRICE formula of treatment (protection, relative rest [functional progression as weight bearing permitted—proprioceptive focus], ice [as the modality of choice], compression, elevation [to assist with control of swelling]).

Unfortunately, he did not respond as anticipated and continued to have pain with weight bearing. During the third week, an additional "navicular view" and CT scan were performed. The impact injury to the dome of the talus was now appreciated. Importantly, most ankle sprain patients can be treated effectively without radiographic assessment as long as no proximal or specific bone tenderness is present. But when a patient does not respond as expected (return to weight bearing and activities of daily living within a few days), additional assessment may be required.

 ## REFERENCES

Inman, V. T. (1976). *Joints of the ankle.* Baltimore: Williams Wilkins.

Stiell, I. G, McKnight, R. D, & Greenberg, G. H, et al. (1994). *Implementation of the Ottawa Ankle Rules. JAMA, 271,* 827–832.

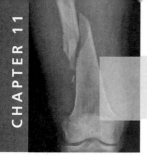

CHAPTER 11

Long Bone Fractures

The appendicular skeletal structures include a set of long bones for both the upper and lower extremities. The special functions associated with these structures provide unique fracture and, thus, healing patterns. Since the lower extremity is weight bearing, specific approaches to fracture management which allow some level of early weight bearing have evolved to better minimize the secondary changes associated with immobilization and a non–weight-bearing status. As a general rule, lower extremity management is all about function (enable return to weight bearing and thus ambulation), whereas upper extremity management is more likely to include a level of attention to cosmesis. The long bones each have inherent patterns of loading related to their individual roles, and thus have specific patterns of injury. These will be addressed in each section of this chapter, and we have chosen primarily to discuss fractures of the shafts of these long bones with the other chapters presenting those which include the articular portion of the bone.

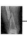 LONG BONE BIOLOGY AND FUNCTION

The long bones are designed to allow placement of the hand in space for function or movement of the body (ambulation) through the transmission and support of weight-bearing loads. These bones can be described in a variety of ways but can easily be perceived as specifically shaped (slightly bent) polyvinyl chloride (PVC) (cortical bone) pipes, firmly packed with dense clay (cancellous bone), and the ends of which have special smooth surfaces (articular covering) to allow them to be joined one to another. These structures receive "pure" loading (application of force) in four ways: tension, compression, bending, and torsion. Fractures are thus linked to each of these loading types: tension—avulsion injury, often soft tissue to bone; compression—compressed or impacted fractures; bending—transverse fractures; torsion—spiral fractures. Importantly, they may also have combination loading which provides combined patterns of fracture resulting in oblique or oblique and transverse fractures. Displacement and whether the skin is intact are then added in the final fracture description. The radiographic presentation then is often very well predicted by the injury mechanism with the type and direction of load and the magnitude as well as velocity, all playing a role in the fracture (Greathouse, 1998) (Figures 11–1 to 11–6).

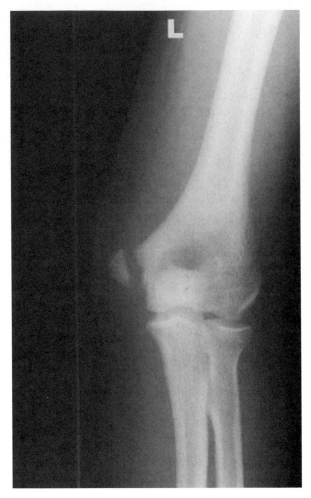

Figure 11–1 Avulsion fracture of medial epicondyle. Tension loading from musculotendinous units can separate the bony attachment point from the main portion of the bone to result in an avulsion fracture.

In reading the radiographs of long bone fractures, the importance of A (alignment) of the A-B-C progression is very significant. Alignment is critical as maintenance of length and positional ability must be preserved as much as possible for optimal functional outcomes. The clinician must appreciate the slight convexity or curvature inherent in many of these bones to avoid alterations or malalignment which may impact function and result in early changes associated with the development of arthritis, particularly in the lower extremity (Figures 11–7 and 11–8).

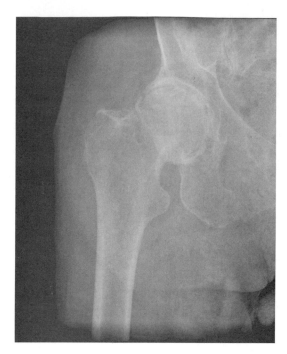

Figure 11–2 Impacted fracture of femoral neck. Beyond capacity compressive loading of the bone can result in an impact fracture. Note the shortening of the femoral neck in this radiograph.

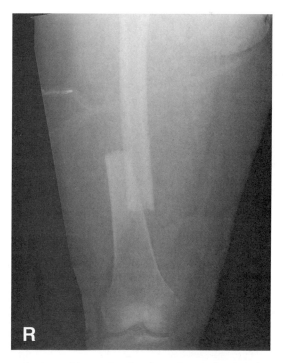

Figure 11–3 Transverse fracture of femur. Bending forces imposed on long bones will typically result in a transverse fracture line across the long axis of the bone as shown on this radiograph.

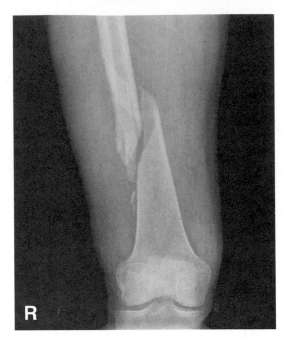

Figure 11–4 Spiral fracture of femur. Torsional loading, perpendicular to the long axis of the bone, is usually the cause of a spiral fracture as it appears in this anteroposterior (AP) radiograph.

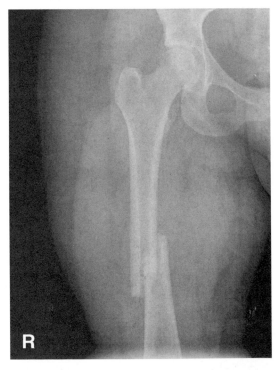

Figure 11–5 Oblique fracture of femur. This AP radiograph demonstrates an oblique fracture of the femur. A combination of compressive and bending loads typically cause these fracture orientations.

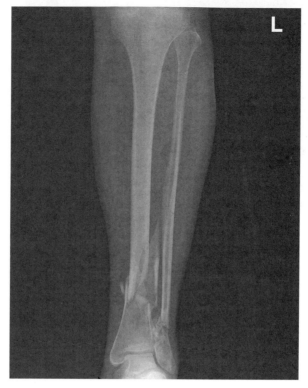

Figure 11–6 Butterfly fracture of tibia. A so-called butterfly fracture occurs from compression and bending forces. This fracture is described by a central fragment surrounded on each side by two other large fragments.

The norm for lower extremity fracture management is to gain and maintain reduction (appropriate alignment; nonsurgically whenever possible) and allow early partial weight bearing to facilitate a healing response while also minimizing the negative effects of disuse. As a general rule, 6 to 8 weeks of protection—reduction, maintenance of reduction (e.g., cast, splint, orthosis); limited—protected partial weight bearing and maintenance of joint ranges of motion whenever possible provide the basic tenets of care for the lower extremity long bone fracture. The upper extremity presents it own set of challenges. Since weight bearing is not an upper extremity functional task, most methods of nonsurgical management do not provide a stimulus for healing but rather, in reality, provide limited control or even distraction after reduction. Thus, 10 to 12 weeks of fracture management is the rule. Although both the leg and forearm increase this challenge, the forearm is particularly difficult because of the numerous rotations and soft tissue attachments which may pull the proximal or distal portion of the bones out of alignment during treatment. This has led to many forearm fractures being surgically fixated (open reduction with internal fixation, ORIF) via plates and screws (Figures 11–9 and 11–10).

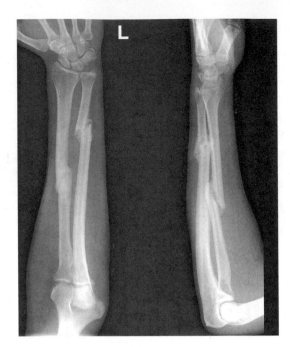

Figure 11–7 Malalignment of upper extremity fractures. In these images of healing fractures of the radius and ulna, suboptimal reduction has occurred. In the AP image, malalignment of the ulnar fracture is particularly evident with effects occurring at the ulnomeniscotriquetral articulation. In the lateral view, the telescoping of the oblique fracture of the radius is demonstrated with resultant shortening, also affecting the wrist mechanics. This patient's chief complaint at the time of presentation of these radiographs was wrist pain, which is possibly due to altered mechanics from the poor fracture alignment.

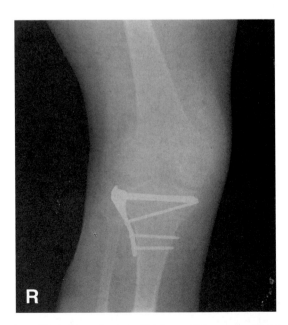

Figure 11–8 Valgus from tibial plateau fracture. This image taken approximately 2 years following a lateral tibial plateau fracture reveals valgus deformity despite the internal stabilization. Residual deformity, often progressing with subsequent degenerative changes, is relatively common in tibial plateau fractures. The alignment and mechanical function of the lower extremity is often increasingly affected.

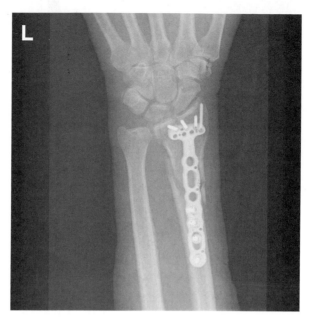

Figure 11–9 ORIF of distal radius fracture. This image demonstrates an internal fixation device being used to stabilize the fragments of a severely comminuted distal radius fracture.

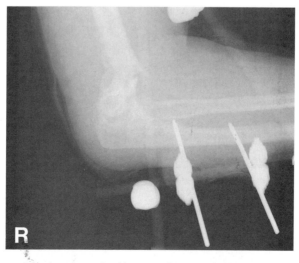

Figure 11–10 External fixation about distal humerus fracture. This lateral view radiograph shows an external fixation device being used to stabilize around a severely comminuted distal humerus fracture. Direct fixation of the fractures was not attempted in this case because of the size, location, and number of fragments. The frame for the external fixator is essentially radiolucent and barely visible in this radiograph.

The key elements related to the treatment of long-bone fractures again relate to the special functional requirements of these structures. Lower extremity fractures have the advantage of weight bearing to facilitate healing but also the challenge of not allowing too much weight bearing too soon and thus refracturing the bone. The upper extremity fractures take longer to heal and have numerous soft tissues applying loads which may create malalignment during fracture management.

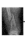 ## ADDITIONAL READING

Anderson, J. (2003). *An atlas of radiography for sports injuries*. New York: McGraw-Hill.

Anderson, J., Read, J. W., & Steinweg, J. (2007). *Atlas of imaging in sports medicine*. New York: McGraw-Hill.

 ## REFERENCES

Greathouse, J. (1998). *Radiographic positioning procedures*. Vol. 1. Albany, New York: Delmar Publishers.

Grey, M. L., & Ailinani, J. M. (2003). *CT & MRI pathology: A pocket atlas*. New York: McGraw-Hill Professional.

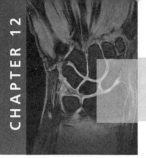

CHAPTER 12

A Primer of "Reading" an Image

RADIOGRAPHY

One of the challenges for becoming comfortable with radiology is the expected or norm for reading and, thus, interpreting a "plain film," whether hard copy or digital. Importantly, in this text we have used the term radiograph to describe what has traditionally been referred to as a plain film (single plane—plain radiographic image)—today this is more typically a digital form but representing the previous image. By convention, the film is placed on a view box or the digital image is oriented on the monitor as if the person were in the anatomic position (facing toward the reader). This allows the reader to have a relatively constant orientation providing an expected presentation and enhancing the ability to perceive the alteration from the norm to be more obvious. Shadows, image magnifications/distortions (size/shape: elongation or foreshortening related to beam orientation and position of bone and distances to film), and overlapping structures thus are seen in their expected positions and the observer is able to concentrate on seeing the abnormal.

Radiographers have agreed to place L (left) or R (right) anatomic markers onto the film to indicate whether the image is of a right or left extremity or side of body. A common novice error is to orient the image to be able to read the R/L designation rather than placement of the image in the anatomic position as the markers will often be placed onto open space and not related to image orientation (e.g., anteroposterior [AP], posteroanterior [PA]) (Figures 12–1 and 12–2). When looking at an extremity, therefore, the image should be placed upright as seen in the anatomic position, except for the hand and foot which are normally placed with the digits and toes directed upward. Additional markers are sometimes used including rotational indicators (e.g., internally rotated [INT] and externally rotated [EXT], weight bearing [WTB], inspiration [INS], with weights—as in stress views associated with the acromioclavicular joint) (Greathouse, 1998).

As a general rule, the bony structure that is at a 90-degree angle to the x-ray tube will appear the most clearly defined and least distorted, whereas the more a bone is angled from the beam, the more it becomes distorted. Also, as a general rule, the closer the structure is to the film plate/receptor, the less distortion and greater definition will be perceived. Loss of image clarity or sharpness can also be related to density and contrast (not using the best combination of exposure time and energy). The radiographer carefully controls these exposure parameters to enable optimal viewing

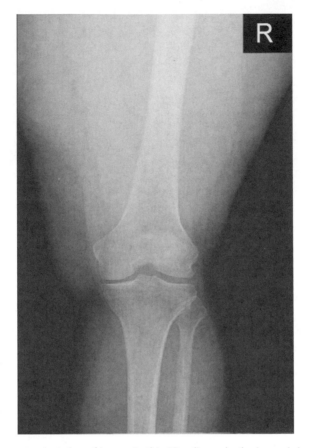

Figure 12–1 Incorrect orientation of image. In this AP radiograph, the image is incorrectly oriented based on reading the identifying label.

properties to be present, particularly attempting to minimize underexposure (too little density and thus appearing whitish) or overexposure (too much density and appearing too dark).

Radiographers always strive to maximize consistency through the orientation of the structure to be exposed, the orientation of the x-ray tube, the position of the "film plate" (often now the receptor), and standardizing distances to enable the peak kilovoltage (kVp—energy) and exposure times then to be relatively consistent. The radiographer creates a book of settings to use with their patients to gain the required views with appropriate contrast with a single set of films. The typical distance of 40 in from tube to film/plate is then the final element in the standardization sequence. Importantly, this process decreases the need for repeat films and thus possible increases in required exposures (repeated films when existing view/plate is not adequate).

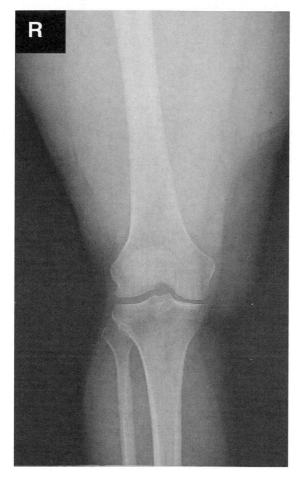

Figure 12–2 Correct orientation of image. The same image is correctly oriented according to the anatomical position in reference to the patient.

 READING THE IMAGE

Once the image is properly displayed, the reader ideally begins with the "set of films" (AP, lateral, oblique, and special views as appropriate) all on the box simultaneously in the old, classic hard copy viewing. This is also known viewing a series , in this case the ankle (typical series is AP, lateral, and either an oblique or mortise view) (Figures 12–3 to 12–6).

A simplistic systematic approach of A-B-C (A, alignment and appearance; B, bone density; C, cortex/consistency) is then applied to initiate the observational and interpretative processes. If the alignment is as expected, the clinician then proceeds to looking at bone density knowing the expected general appearance (cortical is brighter [greater absorption], whereas cancellous is darker [absorbs less as it is less dense]). The final step

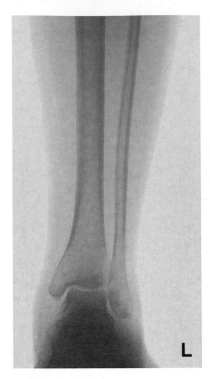

Figure 12–3 A normal-appearing AP view radiograph of the ankle. Note the slight overlap of the tibia and fibula at the distal articulation.

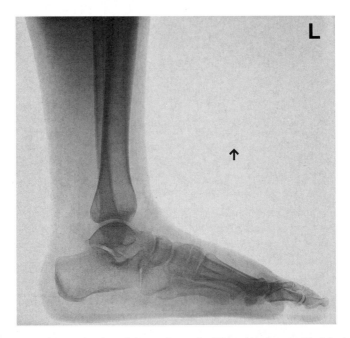

Figure 12–4 A normal-appearing lateral view radiograph of the ankle. Apparent in this view is not only the general osseous alignment but also the joint space of the talocrural joint.

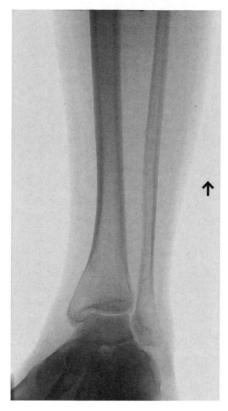

Figure 12–5 The oblique view radiograph allows greater visualization of the malleoli and their surrounding structures.

is to examine the cortex to look for any inconsistencies (breaks) or distortions at the bright edge and also unexpected changes.

Radiography remains the most frequently used imaging modality for initial fracture screening owing to its availability, sensitivity, and economy. The demonstration of altered anatomic position and distinct fracture lines are the basis for the identification of most fractures. A radiologist's report of a radiographic or computerized tomographic (CT) study concerning a fracture typically includes a description of fracture location, position of the bones and bone fragments, and alignment of the bones. In reference to alignment, this typically includes either relative or measured displacement, distraction, overlap, or rotation. If present, the narrative will also include a description of comminution, joint involvement, any evidence of the fracture being open (i.e., tissue gas), foreign bodies, and any suggestion of prior injuries or pre-existing lesions.

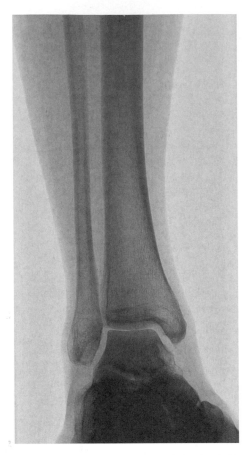

Figure 12–6 In this mortise view radiograph, the overlap of the distal tibia and fibula is eliminated, allowing for better visualization of the talus within the mortise.

 ## RECONSTRUCTED IMAGES

When greater detail than that available by radiography or inspecting soft tissues is of interest, the employment of other imaging modalities is likely. The viewer of CT or magnetic resonance imaging (MRI) sequences and series has a somewhat more complex task than reading radiographs. As reconstructions in virtually any plane are possible with CT and MRI, remarkable anatomic detail in sections or slices can be reproduced in intervals of a few millimeters. Thus, a viewer of CT or MR images must first gain orientation of the images and relevant anatomy. Knowledge of the anatomy at all tissue depths is paramount to have a perspective on the images as being within the realm of normal or abnormal appearance. The viewer must also appreciate the relative sensitivities of the imaging modality to the particular structures of interest. CT, for example, allows for much greater visualization of cortical and trabecular bone and the bony anatomy of joints. Yet, CT does not differentiate all tissue densities well and may not, therefore, identify some soft tissue lesions as well as MRI. Similarly, MRI does not resolve bone mineral well, but the cellular space and fluid content are demonstrated in excellent detail. Thus, MRI can reveal some fractures in superior fashion. Generally, MRI is the modality of choice for assessment of soft tissues, allowing remarkable ability to visualize tissue integrity, continuity, and relative fluid content among sequences. Thus, the viewer of MR images may follow the same basic conceptual framework of examining alignment, bone density or architecture, and cortical signal consistency, along with adding particular attention to the soft tissues. The size, spatial relationships, signal intensities, and detail for tissue continuity and integrity are routinely inspected in detail on MR images.

As described elsewhere (Chapter 1), the imaging sequence or signal measured must be known to be able to interpret the MR images. For example, yellow bone marrow will appear somewhat brighter on T1-weighted images and darker on T2-weighted images (Figures 12–7 and 12–8). Cortical bone, with the high calcium concentration, appears as low signal (darker) on both T1- and T2-weighted images. The presence of increased signal intensity (brightness) on T2-weighted images within or immediately surrounding soft tissues indicates the presence of fluid, often as part of an inflammatory process (Figure 12–9). Other

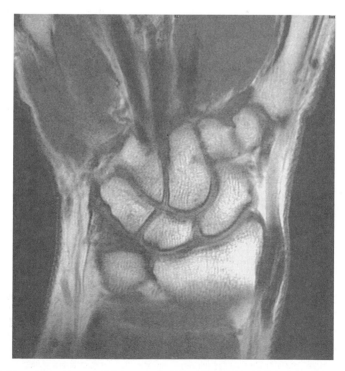

Figure 12–7 T1-weighted image. This is a coronal slice T1-weighted MR image of the wrist. Note the relative signal intensities of the bone and soft tissues.

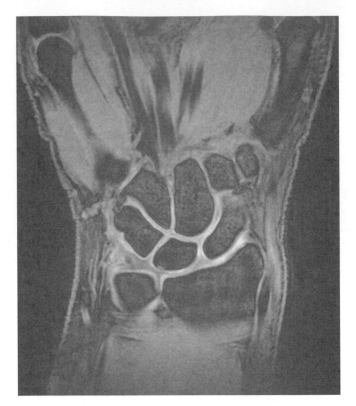

Figure 12–8 T2-weighted image. This coronal slice of the same subject is a T2-weighted MR image. Note the difference in signal intensities compared to the T1-weighted image.

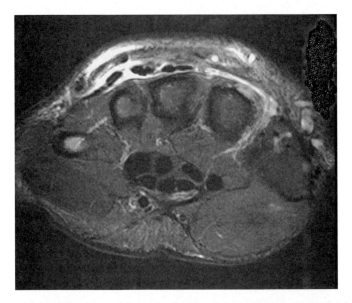

Figure 12–9 Fluid signal. One common criterion for identifying pathologies in T2-weighted imaging sequences is the presence of increased signal intensity indicated the presence of free fluid. In this individual, note the bright signal intensity surrounding the extensor tendons, which is consistent with an inflammatory response.

MRI techniques abound such as fat suppression and fast spin echo to bring about particular effects and contrasts in allowing the image reader greater ability to discriminate the anatomic structures of interest. Additionally, MRI and CT may be completed with the addition of injected contrast agents to increase sensitivity in identifying particular features (Grey, 2003).

The reader of a MRI report from a radiologist will typically find a document of considerable detail. As more anatomy is visible on MRI than radiography, the radiologist will typically describe each tissue type and its appearance in reference to relative normal. Thus, the bony structures will be characterized along with the muscle, tendon, ligament, and cartilaginous/fibrocartilaginous tissues, often in subheadings according to tissue type. Reference is often made to the structural integrity as well as the signal intensity, alterations of which are often associated with ongoing inflammatory or degenerative processes. Narrative is also offered on any space-occupying lesions, hematomas, or other aberrations of normal spatial relationships present. Subsequent or sometimes antecedent to the detailed description, a summary paragraph or itemized list of significant findings is often offered for the reader's convenience.

The enclosed instructional CD provides additional displays and descriptions of the reading/interpreting process along with significant detail. Throughout the text the "expected or normal imaging modalities" are emphasized. In classroom use, we urge the instructor to be certain to use the additional resources of the CD to better provide maximal learning experiences.

ADDITIONAL READING

Anderson, J. (2003). *An atlas of radiography for sports injuries*. New York: McGraw-Hill.

Anderson, J., Read, J. W., & Steinweg, J. (2007). *Atlas of imaging in sports medicine*. New York: McGraw-Hill.

REFERENCES

Greathouse, J. (1998). *Radiographic positioning procedures*. Vol. 1. Albany, New York: Delmar Publishers.

Grey, M. L., & Ailinani, J. M. (2003). *CT & MRI pathology: A pocket atlas*. New York: McGraw-Hill Professional.

INDEX

Note: Page numbers followed by a *t* or *f* indicate that the entry is included in a table or figure.

SOFTWARE AND INFORMATION LICENSE

The software and information on this CD-ROM (collectively referred to as the "Product") are the property of The McGraw-Hill Companies, Inc. ("McGraw-Hill") and are protected by both United States copyright law and international copyright treaty provision. You must treat this Product just like a book, except that you may copy it into a computer to be used and you may make archival copies of the Products for the sole purpose of backing up our software and protecting your investment from loss.

By saying "just like a book," McGraw-Hill means, for example, that the Product may be used by any number of people and may be freely moved from one computer location to another, so long as there is no possibility of the Product (or any part of the Product) being used at one location or on one computer while it is being used at another. Just as a book cannot be read by two different people in two different places at the same time, neither can the Product be used by two different people in two different places at the same time (unless, of course, McGraw-Hill's rights are being violated).

McGraw-Hill reserves the right to alter or modify the contents of the Product at any time.

This agreement is effective until terminated. The Agreement will terminate automatically without notice if you fail to comply with any provisions of this Agreement. In the event of termination by reason of your breach, you will destroy or erase all copies of the Product installed on any computer system or made for backup purposes and shall expunge the Product from your data storage facilities.

LIMITED WARRANTY

McGraw-Hill warrants the physical diskette(s) enclosed herein to be free of defects in materials and workmanship for a period of sixty days from the purchase date. If McGraw-Hill receives written notification within the warranty period of defects in materials or workmanship, and such notification is determined by McGraw-Hill to be correct, McGraw-Hill will replace the defective diskette(s). Send request to:

Customer Service
McGraw-Hill
Gahanna Industrial Park
860 Taylor Station Road
Blacklick, OH 43004-9615

The entire and exclusive liability and remedy for breach of this Limited Warranty shall be limited to replacement of defective diskette(s) and shall not include or extend to any claim for or right to cover any other damages, including but not limited to, loss of profit, data, or use of the software, or special, incidental, or consequential damages or other similar claims, even if McGraw-Hill has been specifically advised as to the possibility of such damages. In no event will McGraw-Hill's liability for any damages to you or any other person ever exceed the lower of suggested list price or actual price paid for the license to use the Product, regardless of any form of the claim.

THE McGRAW-HILL COMPANIES, INC. SPECIFICALLY DISCLAIMS ALL OTHER WARRANTIES, EXPRESS OR IMPLIED, INCLUDING BUT NOT LIMITED TO, ANY IMPLIED WARRANTY OF MERCHANTABILITY OR FITNESS FOR A PARTICULAR PURPOSE.

Specifically, McGraw-Hill makes no representation or warranty that the Product is fit for any particular purpose and any implied warranty of merchantability is limited to the sixty day duration of the Limited Warranty covering the physical diskette(s) only (and not the software or information) and is otherwise expressly and specifically disclaimed.

This Limited Warranty gives you specific legal rights; you may have others which may vary from state to state. Some states do not allow the exclusion of incidental or consequential damages, or the limitation on how long an implied warranty lasts, so some of the above may not apply to you.

This Agreement constitutes the entire agreement between the parties relating to use of the Product. The terms of any purchase order shall have no effect on the terms of this Agreement. Failure of McGraw-Hill to insist at any time on strict compliance with this Agreement shall not constitute a waiver of any rights under this Agreement. This Agreement shall be construed and governed in accordance with the laws of New York. If any provision of this Agreement is held to be contrary to law, that provision will be enforced to the maximum extent permissible and the remaining provisions will remain in force and effect.